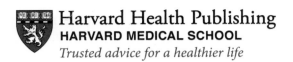

MW00609920

Dear Reader,

Slowly but surely the message is getting out: strength training isn't just for bodybuilders with bulging biceps and rippling abdominal muscles. Like aerobic exercise, it's important for everybody, and everyone should include it as part of a regular exercise program. Studies show that strength training can help prevent or control conditions as varied as heart disease, diabetes, arthritis, and osteoporosis. No matter what your age, it's not too late. The time to start is now, if you want to preserve your quality of life and fight off frailty.

Strength training has many benefits in addition to those listed above. It can tone your muscles and make any sport you play more enjoyable. As you grow older, it can help you perform the tasks of everyday life, such as climbing a flight of stairs, carrying a bag of groceries, putting away a heavy dish in a high cabinet, or even just getting out of a chair.

Recently we've also begun learning about a related concept called power training, which builds both strength and speed. There is overlap between the two, but think of it this way: power training helps you move faster when you walk (allowing you to get across an intersection in a safe amount of time) or react faster (keeping a trip from becoming a fall). The concept of power training was developed in part by our Harvard colleagues Jonathan F. Bean and Walter R. Frontera. It was Drs. Bean and Frontera who wrote the original version of this report, which we would like to recognize and acknowledge here.

Muscles naturally weaken with age—starting in your 30s—so you need to keep working them in order to retain strength and power. The good news is that your investment in exercise can yield quick returns. Studies have found that as little as six weeks of weight workouts can dramatically improve strength, power, mobility, and agility, even in men and women in their 70s, 80s, and 90s.

If you're like many older adults, you may be leery of working out with trainers who are decades younger than you and who don't understand the limitations of aging bodies. If so, this report is for you. In it, you will find two workouts geared to older adults that include both strength and power training. You'll learn how to begin slowly and safely, and what equipment you need to get started. It isn't much. For our easy-to-follow workouts, all you need are sneakers, comfortable exercise clothes, some dumbbells, ankle weights, and a sturdy chair. If you already use weights, you will learn how to step up the pace and keep your routines interesting and fun. Have fun working out. We do!

Sincerely,

Elizabeth Pegg Frates, M.D.
Medical Editor

Michele Stanten
Fitness Consultant

The basics: Strength training, power training, and your muscles

It's one thing to live a long life. It's another to live long and well. The burgeoning field of lifestyle medicine has a perfect description of this goal: "adding not only years to your life, but life to your years." But how do you do that? When it comes to staying healthy and living longer, many people think of eating a heart-healthy diet to help ward off heart attacks, or controlling blood pressure to help prevent strokes. These are indisputably excellent goals. But the truth is, maintaining your muscles should also be high on your list because strong muscles can have a major impact on how well you age.

Your muscles enable you to carry groceries, hoist suitcases into the car, climb stairs, get out of a chair, swing a golf club, and dance the tango. The stronger and more powerful your muscles are, the easier all of these activities and others will be. But neglect your muscles, and it will certainly complicate your life. Weak muscles turn seemingly simple tasks like walking into a chore and are a primary reason that many people lose their independence as they age.

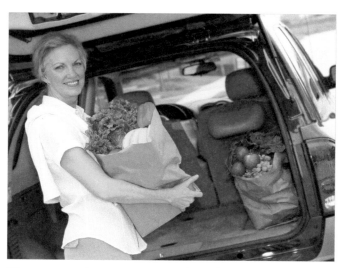

When your muscles are strong, everyday tasks—such as carrying heavy sacks of groceries—are easier. Weak muscles are a leading reason elderly people lose their independence.

Having smaller, weaker muscles doesn't just change the way you look or move. Muscle loss affects the body in many ways. Strong muscles pluck oxygen and nutrients from the blood much more efficiently than weak ones. That means any activity requires less effort from the heart and therefore puts less strain on it. Strong muscles are also better at sopping up sugar in the blood and helping the body stay sensitive to insulin (which helps cells extract sugar from the blood). In these ways, strong muscles can help keep blood sugar levels in check—which in turn helps prevent or control type 2 diabetes.

Strong muscles enhance weight control, too. Muscles fuel your resting metabolic rate—the amount of calories you burn on a daily basis to sustain your breathing, heartbeat, digestion, and other basic bodily functions. The more muscle you have, the higher your metabolic rate is, and the more calories you burn without even trying. This can help prevent age-related weight gain.

Strength and power training are key to keeping your muscles functioning at a high level as you get older. In one study, middle-aged men and women who did just one to three strength workouts a week, totaling less than an hour, were 40% to 70% less likely to have a heart attack or stroke during the 10- to 15-year study than if they did no strength training. And studies of people in their 70s, 80s, and 90s have shown that it's possible to rebuild muscle and strength even at these ages (see "You're never too old to try," page 9).

So exactly what is strength training? What is power training, and how does it differ from strength training? How do your muscles respond to these exercises? You'll find answers to these questions in this chapter. You'll also learn how muscles work and how aging and disuse contribute to the loss of muscle strength and power over the years.

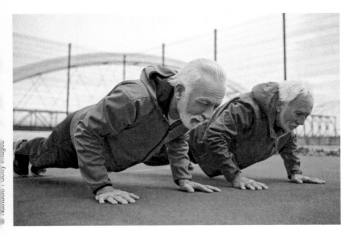

Strength training harnesses resistance to help build muscles. The resistance can come from dumbbells, exercise machines, resistance bands, or your own body weight—as when you perform push-ups.

Strength training: The traditional approach

Strength training is a popular term for exercises that build muscle by harnessing resistance—that is, an opposing force that muscles must strain against. Strength training is sometimes called resistance training, progressive resistance training, or weight training. Resistance can be supplied by your body weight, free weights such as dumbbells and weighted cuffs, elasticized bands, or specialized machines. No matter what kind of resistance you use, putting more than the usual amount of load on your muscles makes them stronger. These exercises can strengthen your bones as well because your muscles are attached to underlying bones. When your muscles contract, they pull on the bones, and this force stimulates the bones to get stronger.

Strength training is not just for 20-somethings in search of buff bodies or bulked-up muscles. While it can certainly reshape a person's silhouette in a pleasing way, it can also boost the strength everyone needs for daily tasks. Just about any activity becomes easier with stronger muscles. So will any sport you enjoy.

Power training: A complementary approach

Another type of training, known as power training, is proving to be just as important as traditional strength training in helping maintain or restore functional abilities—maybe even more important.

As the name suggests, power training is aimed at increasing power, which is the product of both strength and speed, reflecting how quickly you can exert force to produce the desired movement. Thus, faced with a four-lane intersection, you may have enough strength to walk across the street. But can you cross all four lanes of traffic before the light changes? Power, not just strength, can get you from one side to the other safely. Likewise, by helping you react swiftly if you trip or lose your balance, power can actually prevent falls.

Some power moves are just strength training exercises done at a faster speed. Other power routines rely on the use of a weighted vest, which is worn while performing certain exercises that are typically aimed at improving functions such as bending, reaching, lifting, and rising from a seated position. But you don't need a vest to do the power training moves we illustrate in our workouts.

As you age, muscle power declines even more swiftly than strength does—as much as 3.5% a year. So exercises that can produce gains in power become especially important as you get older. That's why some doctors, physical therapists, and personal trainers are now combining the swift moves of power training with slower, more deliberate strength training exercises to reap the benefits of both.

A look at muscles and movement

Before you read about the health benefits of these forms of exercise or try specific exercises, it helps to learn a bit about how your muscles work—and just how strength and power training will affect them.

Your body actually has three types of muscles: cardiac muscle (in the heart), smooth muscles (surrounding hollow organs such as your stomach, intestines, and blood vessels, allowing expansion or contraction of these organs), and skeletal muscles (muscles attached to bone that enable you to move). Of the three, only skeletal muscles are under your conscious control. These are the muscles that strength and power training affect the most directly and the ones we'll be focusing on in this report.

The body boasts more than 600 skeletal muscles that enable you to walk, twist, swing your arms, turn your head, flex your feet, wiggle your toes, and more. These muscles are quite complex. A single muscle has from 10,000 to over a million muscle fibers. Each fiber consists of tiny interlocking strands that contain special proteins, known as contractile proteins, which generate the force for muscle contraction. The fibers are bundled into groups called fasciculi (see Figure 1, below), which enables them to work together. Nerve impulses instruct muscles how to move. A grouping of one nerve and its corresponding muscle fibers is called a motor unit.

Most skeletal muscles have two main types of muscle fibers—slow-twitch (also called type I) and fast-twitch (also called type II). Different types of activity tend to emphasize one or the other.

- Slow-twitch fibers are the prime movers during low- to moderate-intensity endurance activities, such as walking, swimming, biking, or jogging. These fibers are called upon first for most activities, and they can keep acting for long periods.
- Fast-twitch fibers churn out more force than slow-twitch ones, but they are more quickly exhausted. They are recruited for short bouts of sprinting, jumping, or scrambling up a hill.

Perhaps not surprisingly, classic strength training tends to develop primarily the slow-twitch fibers, while power training—with its bursts of faster movement—develops the fast-twitch ones. In practice, however, you use both to varying degrees in almost any activity requiring movement. Take something as mundane as washing the dishes. The slow-twitch fibers act during most of the slow-paced activity of scrubbing, rinsing, and drying. But when you reach overhead to put away a heavy dish, the fast-twitch fibers are recruited because you are doing something that requires a more intense burst of power. The combination of strength training and power training helps keep both types of muscle fibers functioning at their best.

Figure 1: An in-depth look at muscle

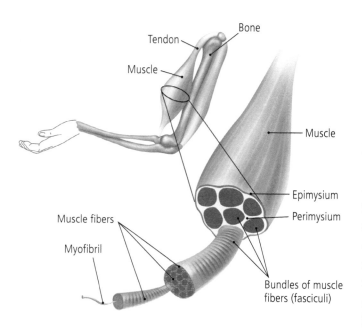

Muscles may seem like simple structures, but they are highly complex.

On the outside, they are covered in connective tissue known as the epimysium and joined to bone by cords of tissue called tendons.

On the inside, they contain small bundles of muscle fibers, known as fasciculi, which allow the fibers in any given bundle to work together in an organized fashion. Each bundle is sheathed in connective tissue, known as the perimysium. In turn, each muscle fiber consists of hundreds to thousands of tiny, interlocking strands called myofibrils. Myofibrils are divided into a series of repeating segments called sarcomeres (not shown), which are considered the contracting unit of skeletal muscle. Within sarcomeres are bands of contractile proteins, called myofilaments (not shown), that generate force for the contraction. Also inside muscle fibers, you will find glycogen (sugar) and fat stores that provide energy for muscle contraction.

Muscles at work

Strength and power training push muscles beyond their usual capacity. Muscles grow in response, because exercise increases the production of new muscle protein. When this cycle occurs repeatedly, muscles become stronger, muscle mass increases, and muscles may become visibly larger, particularly in men. (Women can develop more shapely arms and legs, but they are unlikely to develop big, bulky muscles unless they spend hours a day in the gym, because they don't have enough testosterone for that.) Interestingly, even if there is no visible change in muscle size, strength and power training enhance

Table 1: Know your muscles

A well-rounded strength training program works all the major muscle groups. These are the major muscle groups in your body and the actions and tasks they perform. The workouts in this Special Health Report will ensure that you train all of these key muscles.

BODY PART	MUSCLE	ACTION	EXAMPLE
Shoulders and arms	Deltoid	Moves your entire arm at the shoulder joint	Waving arm overhead
	Biceps	Bends your arm at the elbow joint	Raising a glass to drink
	Triceps	Extends your arm at the elbow joint	Pushing up a window
	Rotator cuff	Rotates arm	Throwing a ball
Back	Trapezius	Moves shoulder and shoulder blade	Shrugging your shoulders
	Rhomboid	Moves shoulder blade	Starting a lawnmower
	Latissimus dorsi	Pulls the arm down	Pulling down a window
	Erector spinae	Extends spine	Standing tall
Front of torso	Rectus abdominis	Bends torso	Sitting up in bed
	Internal and external obliques	Rotate torso	Dancing the twist
Hips, buttocks, and legs	Gluteus maximus	Extends your leg behind you	Standing up from a chair
	Quadriceps	Extends your lower leg at the knee joints	Kicking a ball
	Hamstrings	Pull your heel toward your buttock	Running
	Gastrocnemius and soleus	Point your toes	Rising up onto your toes
	Anterior tibialis	Pulls toes toward shin	Tapping your foot

the ability of the nervous system to activate muscles, enabling you to lift heavier objects and react more quickly.

To allow both a given action and its opposite—to bend your arm and straighten it, for example—muscles work together in pairs, known as agonists and antagonists. The muscle that delivers most of the force needed for a specific movement is called an agonist. To help control the speed and force of the movement and prevent injury, an antagonist works in opposition to the agonist. So, as you walk up stairs, the quadriceps muscles on the fronts of your thighs act as agonists, while the hamstring muscles at the backs of your thighs work as antagonists, helping you to move in a controlled and fluid way. This synergistic relationship is the reason you need to exercise both muscles; otherwise, you will create an imbalance in strength that can increase your chances of being injured. The workouts in this report work all of the major muscle groups for proper muscular development. (Table 1, above,

lists the major muscles and the types of actions they perform.)

Although it's common to think that muscles do nothing more than contract and relax, it's actually more complicated than that. Muscles engage in three types of contractions, all of which you will use in our workouts.

- **Concentric contraction** occurs when muscles shorten while applying the force needed to move bones at a joint. When people think of using their muscles, this is usually what comes to mind—for example, flexing an arm to show off the biceps muscle in the upper arm. Another example of a concentric contraction of the biceps is bending your arms to lift a bag of groceries up to the kitchen counter.

- **Eccentric contraction** occurs when muscles lengthen while applying the force to move bones. This type of action is necessary to help you control a movement—for example, lowering your grocery bag gently rather than simply letting it drop. In this case, the biceps muscle remains actively engaged, even though it is stretching out again. Eccentric strength is especially important for maintaining balance.

- **Isometric (static) contraction** creates force, too, but muscles don't shorten or lengthen much, and bones do not move at joints. If you push against a wall, for example, or try to lift an object that is far too heavy for you, you'll feel your arm muscles tense, but since your muscles can't generate enough force to lift the object or shift the wall, they do not change in length.

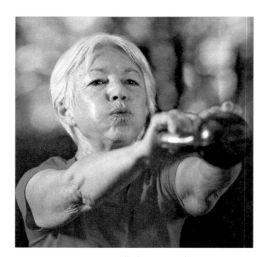

As you age, you naturally lose muscle mass—as much as 4 to 6 pounds of muscle per decade, unless you engage in regular strength training.

Both concentric and eccentric contractions are central to strength and power training, but in different proportions. To build strength, the concentric and eccentric phases of exercises should be of equal length. For example, you'll take the same amount of time to lift a dumbbell (concentric contraction of the biceps) as you will to lower it (eccentric contraction of the biceps). However, to build power, you'll need to make the concentric phase faster—lifting quickly and lowering slowly.

Even though isometric contractions produce little to no movement, they are also effective for building strength. For example, the standing side bridge (page 35) is an isometric exercise, in which muscles throughout much of the body work to hold the body in position. This can help you to stand tall for longer and better maintain your balance. Isometric exercises are also useful when you wish to limit movement, such as when your joints hurt or are inflamed.

Age and muscle loss

As the years pass, muscle mass in the body generally shrinks, and strength and power decline. The process begins earlier than you might think. Sarcopenia—defined as age-related muscle loss—can begin at around age 35 and occurs at a rate of 1% to 2%

a year for the typical person. After age 60, it can accelerate to 3% a year. The loss may be mild, moderate, or severe—or muscles can remain in the normal range. But on average, adults who don't do regular strength training can expect to lose 4 to 6 pounds of muscle per decade. (And most people don't see the number on the scale going down, which means they are replacing that muscle with fat.) Fast-twitch fibers, which provide bursts of power, are lost at a greater rate than slow-twitch fibers, which means you're not only growing weaker but also getting slower.

Weak muscles hasten the loss of independence, putting everyday activities out of reach—activities such as walking, cleaning, shopping, and even dressing. They hinder your ability to cope with and recover from an illness or injury. Disability is 1.5 to 4.6 times higher in older people with moderate to severe sarcopenia than in those with normal muscle mass. Weak muscles also make it harder to balance properly when moving or even standing still—and loss of power compounds the problem. Perhaps it's not surprising that one in every three adults ages 65 and older falls each year. Some of these falls can have dire consequences, including bone fractures, admittance to long-term care facilities, and even death from complications. According to the CDC, these spills lead to more than 800,000 hospitalizations a year. But strength and power training can help. People with stronger muscles are less likely to fall and, when they do take a tumble, less likely to sustain a serious injury.

Loss of muscle strength and mass aren't the only factors that contribute to age-related declines in function and mobility. Mitochondria—the energy-producing "power plants" inside cells—decrease in number and efficiency. Similarly, the nerve-signaling system that recruits muscle fibers for tasks deteriorates with age and lack of use.

While it's tempting to attribute all of these

changes to aging alone, disuse of muscles plays a bigger role than many people suspect. Studies suggest that strength and power training can help reverse these effects and restore muscle function.

Age and intermuscular fat

Research has identified another potential culprit in age-related weakness and disability: fat. The Health, Aging, and Body Composition study (commonly called the Health ABC study) revealed that people who have a greater amount of fat between their muscle fibers might be more likely to experience mobility problems.

The location of the fat is a key factor: the fat normally found *inside* muscle fibers (intramuscular fat) provides fuel for exercising muscles, but fat that accumulates *between* muscle fibers (intermuscular fat, like what you see in a marbled slice of beef) seems to have harmful consequences, contributing to insulin resistance, for example. Not surprisingly, the amount of intermuscular fat tends to increase with age, as weight creeps up. Recent research suggests that the more intermuscular fat you have, the greater your risk of disability, even if you are maintaining your muscle mass.

The good news is that intermuscular fat responds well to a good diet and regular exercise. One small study published in the journal *Gerontology* supported the theory that even in your 80s, you can reduce the amount of fat infiltration in your muscles. In the study, 13 men and women ages 65 to 83 performed resistance training for 24 weeks, stopped the training for 24 weeks, and then resumed it for 12 weeks. After they suspended their routines in the middle phase of the study, the amount of fat in their muscles increased. When they took up their training again, it decreased, even though there was no change in the size of the muscles. More studies are under way to examine how the extent of fat infiltration in muscles affects function and the progression of certain health problems, such as knee osteoarthritis.

All of these factors provide some pretty powerful reasons to take up strength and power training. The next chapter delves into specific health-related benefits of these forms of exercise, besides simply stemming declines in muscle function. ◗

What strength and power training can do for you

You've probably heard it all your life: exercise is good for you. Hundreds of studies have demonstrated the truth of this statement. Regular exercise lowers your risks for serious health problems, such as heart disease, type 2 diabetes, high blood pressure (hypertension), and certain forms of cancer. What's more, as you advance toward old age, it preserves independence by helping you retain the ability to carry out tasks and chores for yourself. And as an added reward, it can help trim your silhouette.

While most exercise studies have focused on aerobic (cardio) activity—exercise like walking, running, or swimming that increases heartbeat and breathing rate for a sustained period—a growing number of studies have shown that strength and power training deliver significant health benefits as well (see "Benefits at a glance," below left). The more muscle you have and the stronger your muscles are, the more benefits you'll get—even from your cardio workouts. When your muscles are strong, you can go faster and last longer.

This chapter describes some of the primary health benefits of these forms of exercise, starting with power training, which is newer to the scene and has been studied less extensively.

Health benefits of power training

Football players, high jumpers, and other athletes have long used power training, particularly with weighted vests, to help improve performance. Many studies have documented not only improvements in performance with power training, but also reductions in injuries.

For non-athletes, there aren't as many studies on power training, but research in this area is growing and has already yielded promising results. The documented benefits include preventing falls, preserving and enhancing physical functioning, and improving quality of life. As this implies, power training in older adults can help stem the progression from gradual impairment to limited daily functioning and then to outright disability. A number of studies have confirmed that power training can make everyday tasks more manageable. While strength training is beneficial, power training appears to be even more effective for improving your ability to accomplish daily tasks, according to the latest research.

Power training could even help with one daily task that you might not think would improve with exercise—driving. Researchers found that older adults (ages 70 and above) who did 12 weeks of power training leg exercises could brake faster in a driving simu-

Benefits at a glance

While practically any regular exercise promotes good health, here's a quick summary of what strength and power training can do for you.

- strengthen muscles
- strengthen bones
- prevent falls and fractures by improving balance and preserving the ability to correct missteps
- improve cholesterol levels
- help control blood sugar
- improve the body's ability to draw oxygen and nutrients from the bloodstream for growth, energy, and repair
- help keep weight within a healthy range

- improve blood flow, so the heart doesn't have to work as hard
- prevent or ease lower back pain
- relieve arthritis pain and expand range of motion in joints
- raise confidence, brighten mood, and help fight mild to moderate depression
- ward off loss of independence by keeping muscles strong enough for routine tasks.

You'll learn more about many of these benefits in this chapter.

You're never too old to try

We all want to maintain our mobility and independence as long as possible. Exercise—including strength and power training—can help you achieve that goal. While senior programs often focus on very light exercise and stretching regimens, research shows that it is not necessary or even especially helpful to limit your exercise in this way. Even people hobbled by serious conditions, such as severe frailty, can do strength and power training using the simple exercises in this report, such as biceps curls (page 34) and chair stands (page 32).

One study found that for some adults 80 and older, 10 weeks of strength training allowed them to forgo a walker in favor of a cane. A review of 11 studies of seniors, ages 61 to 91, found that strength training two or three times a week for six weeks to a year improved mobility, walking speed, and balance and reduced the risk of falling.

You can even do power training in your 90s. In one study, researchers tested 24 frail people who were in their late 80s and early 90s and living in a nursing home. Half of the group followed a 12-week exercise program, consisting of power, balance, and gait training, while the other

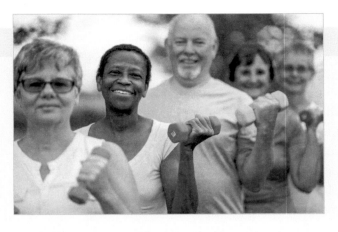

half did traditional mobility exercises for this age group. Ninety percent of the power training group stuck with the program, suggesting that the routines were doable and there were few injuries. Those seniors increased strength and power, performed everyday functions (such as getting in and out of a chair and walking) more easily, lowered their incidence of falls, and reduced intermuscular fat. In contrast, the other group showed no improvements or, worse, experienced further declines in performance. So no matter how old you are, start strength and power training now, and you'll get benefits.

lation than older adults who did 12 weeks of regular strength training exercises or stretching exercises.

There may also be benefits for people with certain health problems. One small study tested three types of exercise—strength training, power training, and stretching—on people with osteoarthritis of the knee. After 12 weeks of exercise, participants in all three groups had better function and less pain, but those in the power training group registered the greatest gains in strength, power, and walking speed. (A second small study found no gains in speed, but did confirm reductions in pain and improvements in tasks of daily living.)

Not surprisingly, these gains can translate into a better quality of life. For a study published in *Health Quality of Life Outcomes*, researchers randomly assigned 45 older adults to a strength training group, a power training group, or a control group that performed no exercise. Both the exercise groups reported improvements in physical functioning compared with those who did no exercise, but only the power training participants reported greater satisfaction with their quality of life.

Health benefits of strength training

Scientists have long known that strength training has a positive impact on your body. Conditions as varied as back pain, heart disease, arthritis, osteoporosis, diabetes, obesity, and insomnia can be partly managed by strength training and other exercise regimens. But what is the relative importance of strength training versus aerobic workouts? Relatively few large, long-term studies have examined this question.

Some things are clear, however. Strong muscles never sleep. Studies have found that strength training can increase your metabolic rate (the rate at which your body converts energy stores into working energy) by up to 15%. This lets you burn more calories, even while you're sitting or sleeping. Coupled with the calories you use up during strength training workouts, this increase in metabolism may help you stay at a healthy weight or even lose some weight, provided you're eating right.

A solid line of research shows that shaving off as little as 10% of excess weight pays big health dividends. Because obesity factors into many health problems—including high blood pressure, heart disease, gallbladder disease, arthritis, diabetes, and certain cancers—that's an investment that keeps giving back.

Strength training also counteracts unhealthful changes in your body composition. As muscle tissue shrinks with disuse and age, most people replace lost muscle with fat. In addition to creating more rolls of flab, this trade raises the risk for type 2 diabetes. Muscle tissue is better than fat at controlling blood sugar and reducing insulin resistance (the primary cause of type 2 diabetes). In addition, strength training can help peel away an unhealthy girdle of abdominal fat, reducing your risk for heart disease and stroke—and even helping you to live longer. When researchers looked at the exercise habits of men and women ages 65 or older, they found that those who did strength training were 46% less likely to die during the 15-year study than those who did no strength training.

In this chapter, we outline some other ways in which strength training improves specific health conditions, possibly even reducing the need for medications (see "A potent prescription: Exercise," below left). We've also included tips to consider before you embark on a workout if you have one of these conditions.

Easing arthritis pain

Done properly, strength training can make a significant difference to people with many types of arthritis. That's why both the Arthritis Foundation and the CDC recommend it.

But arthritis pain presents a difficult dilemma for many people—at least at the outset. On one hand, strengthening muscles helps support and protect joints. And exercise, including strength training, helps ease pain, stiffness, and possibly swelling; enhances the range of motion in many joints; and trims excess weight that harms joints. On the other hand, it can be difficult to start weight training if you have arthritis. Muscles that have not been exercised may be weak and less able to support joints properly. As a result, range of motion, already limited by arthritis, is further restricted. But while it may be difficult to strength train initially, doing so typically pays dividends ultimately by improving joint function—provided you begin with light weights or low resistance to avoid joint damage.

One of those dividends—better range of motion—is welcome news if you find you no longer have the flexibility to perform basic tasks such as bending down to tie your shoe. In a randomized controlled study of 32 older men, after 16 weeks of workouts, men doing strength training alone or combined with cardiovascular training had significantly more range of motion in all five of the joints tested compared with men who remained inactive. Among those doing just cardiovascular activities, range of motion improved in only one of the joints that were tested.

A potent prescription: Exercise

Medications are well-proven lifelines for millions of people, but some physicians routinely write prescriptions for exercise as well. Conditions such as heart disease, arthritis, osteoporosis, diabetes, and insomnia can be partly managed—and sometimes partly prevented—by strength training and other exercise regimens.

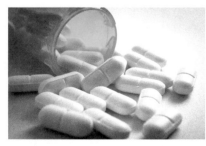

Regular exercise sometimes makes it possible to cut back on medications, but talk to your doctor before adjusting your dose.

In some cases, regular exercise may make it possible for you to cut back on, or even eliminate, certain medications. In this way, choosing an exercise prescription can sidestep or help squelch potentially unpleasant side effects that typically occur when you need higher dosages of medications or multiple drugs. Of course, before discontinuing any medication or changing the dose, talk with your doctor about the role that exercise can play in your treatment needs.

Strength training also has considerable spillover benefits. While you might choose it for a specific reason—for instance, to help unfreeze joints locked up by arthritis—you may find that your regular workouts help you manage or prevent a host of other health problems. No single pill can make the same boast.

Strength training can also ease pain and improve quality of life. In one study, older women who had either knee osteoarthritis or a knee replacement did strength training twice a week for 13 weeks. By the end of the study, the women had improved their ability to walk, climb stairs, and balance. A study in *Arthritis Care Research* also found that people with knee osteoarthritis who did power training reduced pain and improved their ability to function. (If you've had a joint repair or replacement, see "A warning for people with joint repairs or replacements," at right, for some precautions.)

In osteoarthritis, the cartilage that cushions the joints gradually wears away. Studies suggest that greater quadriceps strength protects against this cartilage loss in the knee, since those muscles protect the joint; without strong quadriceps, the joint bears the brunt of the impact, especially when walking or bearing weight. But when strong muscles contract, they take pressure off the joints. Because excess weight worsens osteoarthritis, strength training's ability to help you control your weight is important, too.

People with rheumatoid arthritis can also benefit from strength training, since muscle weakness is common among those with this illness. Multiple studies show improvements in function and strength and reductions in pain and disability following strength training programs. A key to reaping long-term benefits, though, was consistency with the training program.

Tips for people with arthritis

- Have a physiatrist, physical therapist, or certified personal trainer who has experience working with people with arthritis help you design and adapt an exercise program that will work for you. Your exercise program should include strength training, flexibility activities that enhance range of motion, and aerobic activities that avoid further stress on joints, such as water exercise and use of elliptical machines. If necessary, an occupational therapist may be able to suggest splints or assistive devices that will make exercise less painful.
- Schedule workouts for times of the day when your medications are working well, in order to reduce

A warning for people with joint repairs or replacements

If any joints in your body have been surgically repaired or replaced, certain exercises may do more harm than good. If you have had a hip repair or replacement, for example, talk with your surgeon before engaging in lower-body strength training. Usually, people are advised not to cross their legs or do any activity that bends the hips farther than a 90° angle for a certain amount of time after surgery. You may need to modify certain exercises—such as squats and hip rotation stretches—or substitute different exercises into your routine. Don't write off strength training, though: choosing the right exercises for you and doing them properly will help strengthen muscles that support the joint. Your doctor will help you determine the exercises that are best for you.

inflammation and pain. For example, avoid morning workouts if stiffness is at its worst then.
- Before exercise, apply heat to sore joints or take a warm shower or bath. After exercise, cold packs may be helpful.
- If you have rheumatoid arthritis or another form of inflammatory arthritis, include gentle stretching in your warm-up. Inflammation weakens the tendons that tie muscle to bone, making them more susceptible to injury. Remember to use slow movements during your warm-up, and gradually extend your range of motion.
- If you have rheumatoid arthritis, decrease the amount and intensity of your workouts when your condition flares up to reduce inflammation, pain, and fatigue. When it calms down, you can exercise more. Staying active with frequent rest breaks tends to help more than long periods spent in bed.
- Exercise within a comfortable range of motion. If an entire exercise causes significant pain, stop doing it! Discuss other options with your trainer or physical therapist.
- Generally, you should avoid doing strength or power training with actively inflamed joints, at least until the inflammation eases. In some cases, water workouts may be a better choice than strength or power training.

Reducing heart disease risk

Five of the modifiable risk factors for cardiovascular disease—inactivity, high cholesterol, high blood pressure, excess body fat, and diabetes—respond in varying degrees to strength training. Despite this, for years physicians were reluctant to suggest strength training to anyone with a heart condition, fearing it could be dangerous or even fatal. That's no longer the case—at least not across the board. Recommendations from the American Heart Association now suggest that resistance training is safe and beneficial for low-risk cardiac patients, such as people who don't have heart failure, symptoms of angina (chest pain) during exercise testing, or severe heart rhythm abnormalities.

Many cardiologists are willing to extend that exercise prescription further. People who have had heart attacks may start strength training as little as three weeks afterward if their cardiologists recommend it, rather than waiting the more conservative four to six months proposed in older guidelines. In some cases, people suffering from heart failure or awaiting heart transplants because of heart failure can benefit from strength training, provided the condition is stable. In any of these situations, you should speak to your doctor before starting any type of exercise program.

An analysis of 12 studies on aerobic exercise or a combination of aerobic exercise and resistance training in people attending cardiac rehabilitation (where a person might go after a heart attack, stroke, or other serious cardiovascular event) also found that strength training should be part of the program for people with heart disease. The researchers noted that the combination routine decreased body fat, increased strength, and improved overall physical fitness more than aerobic training alone.

By rebuilding muscle, strength training not only gives you more strength for daily tasks, but also helps your body pull oxygen and nutrients from the bloodstream more efficiently and lightens the load on your heart. If you do strength training regularly, your heart rate and blood pressure are less likely to soar when you perform daily activities like carrying groceries. Such changes may improve heart failure symptoms such as breathlessness and fatigue, too.

Strength training can also protect you from having a stroke, a medical emergency in which blood flow to the brain is blocked or reduced. It may even help with recovery after a stroke. People who did strength training three to six months after they had a stroke improved muscle strength and power, walking ability, and cognitive skill, according to an analysis of five studies.

Tips for people with heart disease

- Talk with your physician before embarking on a strength training program. If your heart disease is mild or well controlled by medications, odds are good that strength training is safe for you. Ask whether you need a cardiac exercise stress test beforehand and a monitored exercise program initially; if so, your doctor may refer you to a hospital, clinic, or cardiac rehabilitation center.
- Strength training is not advised if you have unstable angina, uncontrolled high blood pressure, an uncontrolled heart rhythm disorder, heart failure that has not been effectively treated, severe heart valve disease, or hypertrophic cardiomyopathy (a condition in which part of the heart enlarges and obstructs blood flow).
- If you have heart failure, get a baseline cardiac exercise stress test before beginning strength training, and start out in a monitored exercise program. Also, allow 10 to 15 minutes of gentle activity to

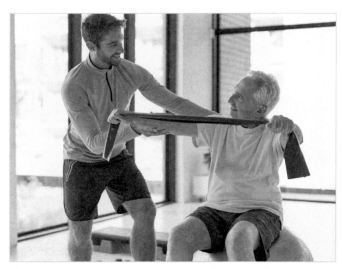

The American Heart Association now says that strength training is safe and beneficial for low-risk cardiac patients, but you may want to start with a monitored program in a clinic or cardiac rehab center.

© PeopleImages | Getty Images

warm up your muscles, lungs, and heart. Initially, work out at low intensity.

- Be sure to keep breathing while lifting and lowering weights. Paradoxically, although you can shave points off your blood pressure reading if you exercise regularly, blood pressure actually goes up *during* exercise—and holding your breath while straining can raise blood pressure to dangerous levels. Counting out loud may help because you can't hold your breath when you're speaking.

- Be aware that many drugs given to help treat heart disease may affect you when you're exercising. Beta blockers, for example, keep heart rate artificially low; that means your pulse is not a good indicator of how vigorously you are exercising. Vasodilators and ACE inhibitors may make you more prone to dizziness from a drop in blood pressure if your post-exercise cool-down is too short. Talk with your doctor about the medications you take. If you work with an exercise professional, be sure he or she understands the potential effects, too.

- If your doctor clears you for strength training, try to choose a supervised program with a certified trainer who understands your condition.

Slowing osteoporosis

A combination of age-related changes, inactivity, and poor nutrition conspire to weaken bones over time (see Figure 2, at right), with bone mass declining at an average rate of 1% per year after age 40. About 10 million Americans have osteoporosis, which is defined by weak and porous bones, and another 44 million are at risk for it. According to the National Osteoporosis Foundation, about half of all women older than 50, and up to one in four men, will break a bone because of osteoporosis. This may happen as the result of a fall or even a far less obvious stress, such as bending over to tie a shoelace.

The effects can be devastating. Hip fractures are usually the most serious. One-fourth of people over the age of 50 who break a hip die within a year from problems related to the broken bone itself or the surgery to repair it. Of those who do survive the hip fracture, many need nursing home care.

Numerous studies have shown that strength and power training can play a role in slowing bone loss, and several show it can even build bone. This is tremendously useful to help offset age-related decline in bone mass, especially among postmenopausal women. Activities that put stress on bones stimulate extra deposits of calcium and nudge bone-forming cells into action. The tugging on bone that occurs during strength and power training (and weight-bearing aerobic exercise like walking or running) provides the stress. The result is stronger, denser bones.

Yet strength and power training has benefits beyond those offered by aerobic weight-bearing exercise. It targets bones of the hips, spine, and wrists, which, along with the ribs, are the sites most likely to fracture. It can help erase another worry, too. Fear of falling can seriously curtail activities of all sorts, espe-

Figure 2: A fragile state

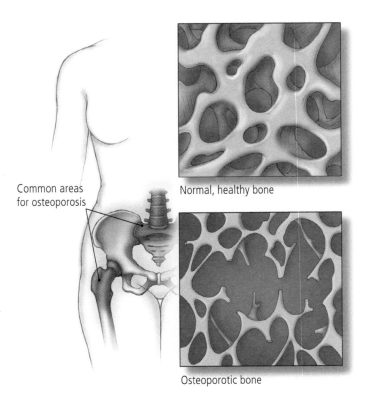

Common areas for osteoporosis

Normal, healthy bone

Osteoporotic bone

Osteoporotic bone is more porous and less dense than healthy bone. The result is bone that is fragile and more vulnerable to breaks. But strength and power training can slow bone loss and even help build bone.

cially among older adults. Resistance workouts—particularly those that include moves emphasizing power and balance—enhance strength and stability. That can boost confidence, encourage you to stay active, and reduce fractures by cutting down on falls.

Tips for people with osteoporosis

- Talk with your doctor before beginning strength training. You may need to adapt certain exercises to make them safer. Initially, it's a good idea to start training with an exercise specialist who works with people with osteoporosis—or to join a program designed for people with osteoporosis—to ensure that you are holding weights correctly and using them safely.

- Research shows that balance exercises significantly reduce falls. And fewer falls can mean fewer broken bones, a major cause of temporary or permanent disability. Several of the exercises in this report can help with balance, including the standing calf raise (page 32), chair stand (page 32), hip extension (page 33), side leg raise (page 38), and thigh raise (page 49).

- Always choose challenging weights that make it somewhat hard to do eight repetitions, and continue to add weight whenever it becomes easy to do 12 repetitions. The forces associated with muscles contracting and relaxing help to prevent bone loss.

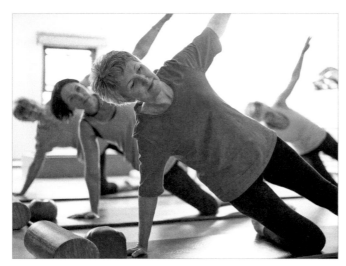

Side bridges can help build core strength, which is essential for everyone, but especially people with osteoporosis. Core strength can help prevent falls that can be devastating if you fracture a hip.

Work with a trainer or physical therapist to help find the right amount of weight that will protect bone without being so heavy that it causes injury.

- Protect your spine. Strength training exercises that help protect the spine and build strong core muscles include the standing side bridge (page 35), side bridge (page 39), bridge (page 38), back extension (page 39), push-up (page 49), and opposite arm and leg raise (page 50). Avoid activities and exercises that require you to twist or bend your spine, especially to lift a weight. This includes bowling, golfing, and even some household tasks. Bend your knees instead of your back when picking something up. Choose abdominal exercises that lift the head and neck just a few inches rather than bringing your trunk to your knees. Avoid free-weight exercises and machines that put added stress on the spine, such as some leg-press machines, leg raises performed lying down, and squats done with weight bars resting on the shoulders.

- Consider trying exercises using a weighted vest, especially if you are a postmenopausal woman (see "How to use a weighted vest," page 46). Studies have shown that progressive training using a weighted vest can increase the development of new bone in women who have already gone through menopause.

- Because power moves improve your ability to recover your balance quickly and avoid falling, they warrant a place in your exercise routine.

Helping manage diabetes

Strength training can reduce your risk of developing diabetes, and if you already have the condition, strength training can help you better control it. Diabetes is a metabolic disorder characterized by high levels of blood sugar (glucose). It occurs when your body doesn't produce enough insulin (type 1 diabetes) or when your body's cells don't respond properly to insulin (type 2 diabetes). Insulin is a hormone that ushers glucose from the bloodstream into cells, where it supplies energy. If there isn't enough insulin or if the cells don't respond appropriately to insulin, too much sugar remains in the blood, damaging tissues throughout the body.

More than 30 million people in the United States have diabetes, and about 12 million of them are older than 65. The vast majority of people with diabetes have type 2. Strength training and other forms of exercise reduce the risk of developing type 2 diabetes, and for those who already have it, reduce the risk of complications by improving blood sugar control. Skeletal muscle serves as a reservoir for glucose, penning up blood sugar not immediately needed for fuel in the form of glycogen and doling it out as necessary. Stronger muscles enable the body to more efficiently sop up circulating blood sugar. Research shows that just one exercise session speeds the rate at which glucose enters the muscles, although that effect dissipates in two to four days unless the activity is repeated.

When it comes to preventing diabetes, regular workouts also help the body remain sensitive to insulin rather than succumbing to the creeping insulin resistance so common among older adults. By burning calories and boosting metabolism, strength training strikes at another potent risk factor for type 2 diabetes: excess weight. A long-term Harvard study published in *The New England Journal of Medicine* attributed about 60% of cases in 85,000 nurses to excess weight. Strength training has also been shown to reduce the unhealthy girdle of fat that encircles the abdomen. This fat layer, which creates an "apple" body shape (as opposed to a "pear" shape from fat on the hips), is linked to insulin resistance and cardiovascular disease. But even if you don't lose weight, you'll still benefit from exercise.

When diabetes does develop, strength training can help control it. One study of older adults with type 2 diabetes found that four months of strength training improved blood sugar control so much that seven out of 10 volunteers were able to reduce their dosage of diabetes medicine. This could have particular resonance for blacks, American Indians, and Hispanics, who are more likely than other Americans to struggle with obesity and diabetes.

One analysis looked at combined data from 47 studies of people with diabetes who worked out for at least 12 weeks. In these studies, the participants' HbA1c levels, which indicate blood sugar control over the previous two to three months, were lower if they engaged in strength training. This held true whether they did strength training alone or also performed aerobic exercise.

Even when insulin is not being produced in normal amounts by the body—as is the case with type 1 diabetes—lowering blood sugar through strength training can reduce the amount of injected insulin a person needs for keeping blood sugar under control.

Tips for people with diabetes

- Talk with your doctor about adjusting your medications before starting a strength training program. Exercise, including strength training, uses glucose, so it may affect the dose of medication you need and maybe even the timing of when you take it.
- Keep carbohydrates like hard candy or glucose tablets with you when you exercise in case your blood sugar drops precipitously, a condition called hypoglycemia. Signs of hypoglycemia include sweating, trembling, dizziness, hunger, and confusion.
- Wear a diabetes bracelet or ID tag and carry phone numbers in case of emergency while exercising.
- Lift challenging loads. Blood sugar control has been shown to improve with high-intensity resistance training. Lighter weights or resistance may not have the same effect.
- Try a power move called the foot roll (see "Foot roll: A power move to help you regain your footing," page 16). One frequent complication of diabetes is dete-

▶ Foot roll: A power move to help you regain your footing

People with diabetes can suffer a complication called peripheral neuropathy, which compromises sensation in the feet. This condition can hamper your balance and make it hard to regain your footing after missteps. (It can also lead to foot ulcers and, ultimately, amputation.) In one study, a six-week program of stretching, strengthening, and balance exercises helped patients with diabetic neuropathy achieve functional improvements. In another, a 12-week program of tai chi helped improve balance and reduce neuropathic symptoms.

According to a small study published in *Archives of Physical Medicine and Rehabilitation*, adding a power move called a foot roll to your workout may also help you respond swiftly when you lose your balance. Stand with your hands holding on to the back of a chair and your feet together. Quickly roll both feet to their outer edges and back again. Do eight to 12 repetitions.

rioration in peripheral nerves, which can diminish sensation in the feet and impair balance. This power move may help you maintain your balance.

Other conditions

Here are a few more ailments that may benefit from regular strength training. (Research on power training's effect on these conditions is still in its infancy.)

Depression. A series of studies suggest regular exercise helps lift mild to moderate depression in some people. There is also evidence that people who are physically active are less likely than those who are sedentary to suffer from depression in the first place.

While early research focused on aerobic activities, studies on strength training's effect on depression are starting to pile up. Two recent analyses drawing on data from dozens of studies and thousands of participants show that strength training reduces depressive symptoms. While the studies didn't look at the reasons why strength training may help, there are some possible explanations. Restoring lost abilities tends to boost confidence and open up new options for pleasurable activities; it may also alleviate dependence on others and fear of falling. Social opportunities offered

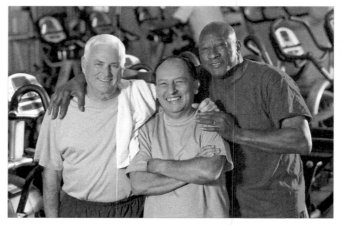

Both aerobic exercise and strength training appear to help lift mild to moderate depression in some people. Restoring lost abilities can boost confidence and open new options for pleasurable activities.

by exercise programs could provide a lift, as well.

Therefore, strength training, alone or mixed with aerobic workouts, may be worth a try in combating mild to moderate depression. One study of 60 older adults with depression found that high-intensity strength training was more effective at reducing depressive symptoms than low-intensity strength training, so choose challenging weights and keep working out regularly. Combining exercise with therapy or with both therapy and medication may prove more successful than exercise alone.

See a doctor or mental health professional if symptoms weigh heavily on you or interfere with daily life. Symptoms of depression include changes in appetite; insomnia or oversleeping; feelings of exhaustion, worthlessness, or inappropriate guilt; and agitation or unusual slowness in thinking, talking, or performing tasks. If you have suicidal thoughts, seek help immediately.

Fibromyalgia. This condition is characterized by widespread musculoskeletal pain, including specific painful areas called trigger points. Fatigue, depression, sleep problems, anxiety, and memory problems are other symptoms. While there is no cure for fibromyalgia, there are options for treating the symptoms, and strength training is one of them. A 2018 review of 22 studies found that just two strength workouts a week could reduce the number of trigger points and pain in general. For example, in a 16-week study included in the review, use of pain medication was lower in the strength training group (41% of participants) compared with the control group (80% of participants) by the end of the study. The review also found that strength training decreased depression and anxiety and improved sleep and quality of life.

Parkinson's disease. Preliminary research points to strength training's possible role in managing the debilitating effects of Parkinson's disease. For example, a small study on Parkinson's found that, compared with a control group engaging in other forms of exercise, patients who performed high-intensity resistance training improved their muscle force and walking speed and scored higher on a quality-of-life questionnaire. Because individuals with Parkinson's often experience slowness in movement, these findings offer hope to them for facilitating activities of daily living.

Down syndrome. People with Down syndrome typically have significantly less strength than unaffected individuals, according to the American College of Sports Medicine, so it's not surprising that lots of strength training studies are being done in this population. What is surprising is the range of benefits to be had. Research has shown strength training to increase strength, improve everyday physical performance, boost immunity, rev up activity levels, and reduce chronic inflammation that can contribute to diabetes and metabolic syndrome in people with Down syndrome. One study found that with 10 weeks of strength training exercises, a small group of individuals with Down syndrome improved their upper-body strength by an average of 42% and their lower-body strength by an impressive 90%. Participants also improved their ability to go down steps and get up from a chair.

Lymphedema. For women suffering from arm swelling after breast cancer surgery, strength training may offer some relief. A study published in *The New England Journal of Medicine* found that of 141 breast cancer survivors who had lymphedema, those who did weight training twice a week for 13 weeks had greater improvements in upper-body strength and a greater reduction of symptoms. In addition, they were no more likely to develop increased limb swelling than those in a group that did not do weight training. These findings call into question the long-held medical view that women who have had breast cancer surgery should avoid stressing the arm for fear that muscle strain could worsen arm swelling. ◖

Getting set up

What you need to get started with strength and power training depends on the activities you choose. You may opt for a program that relies simply on your body weight, or you might choose to use dumbbells or machines designed for strength training. Some people prefer to work out at a gym or take classes, while others value the privacy and convenience of a home workout.

With so many products available, you might need some help sorting through your choices. Table 2 (below) describes major categories of strength training equipment and notes their pros and cons.

Buying basic equipment

Want a good home gym you can easily tuck away? The following will get you started:

- **Dumbbells in a few different weights.** Depending on your current strength, you might start with as little as a set of 2-pound and 5-pound weights or 5-pound and 8-pound weights. Add heavier weights as needed. For buying tips, see "Building smarter dumbbells," page 19.
- **Ankle weights and cuffs with pockets to hold weight bars.** Brands with ½-pound weight bar inserts are best. Look for cuffs that can hold up to at least 5 pounds per leg so you can progress. Depending on the exercises you intend to do, a single ankle cuff worn on one leg at a time may be fine. For the exercises described in this report, you will need only a single cuff.
- **A nonslip exercise mat** (a thick carpet will do in a pinch).
- **A sturdy chair,** preferably with armrests.

Table 2: Choosing strength training equipment

EQUIPMENT	PROS	CONS
Your body weight	• free • always available	• can be hard to increase intensity
Elastic bands or tubes (also called resistance bands or tubes)	• inexpensive • light enough to take anywhere	• difficult to identify the amount of resistance • can snap back at you if not secured properly • become less elastic over time
Free weights (including standard and adjustable weights such as dumbbells or barbells, and ankle or wrist cuffs that hold weight bars)	• fairly inexpensive • good choice at home or at a gym • with free weights, you exercise more muscles, because they are necessary to properly control the weight and achieve good form	• helpful to have initial supervision or to take a class to ensure good form and safe use; good form is important even if weights are light, but becomes even more so with heavier hand weights and barbells • may be hard to sufficiently increase leg weights in order to progress • momentum may make it easier to lift the load
Weight machines (Cybex, Nautilus, Technogym, etc.)	• machine helps ensure good form • easy to add weight as needed • many machines are designed to vary the weight lifted throughout the range of motion of an exercise so that the challenge to the muscle remains optimal • most machines have safety devices	• costly • certain kinds are available only at a gym • best to have initial supervision to ensure you are using the machines safely and properly • momentum may make it easier to lift the load • some machines fail to support or adjust well for women and seniors

- **A set of weight-lifting gloves (optional).** Gloves work well to cushion hands and keep them from slipping on weights.
- **A weighted vest (optional).** This may be useful for some power moves. When shopping for a vest, make sure to look for one that has pockets for adding or removing weight bars, so you can adjust the weight level to suit your body size and strength (see "How to use a weighted vest," page 46). You can find vests online by searching for "weighted vest," or you may be able to find them at a department store, discount store, or sporting goods store. Prices range from about $30 to more than $200.

Investing wisely in large equipment

If you're considering buying large equipment, choose carefully. The Federal Trade Commission (FTC) warns that quite a bit of the equipment being hawked as part of the multibillion-dollar exercise industry doesn't deliver on its promise. Gather enough information to make a good decision before you spend money. The following strategies also apply if you want to buy a home machine (a treadmill, elliptical, or stationary bike, for example) for the aerobic part of your workout.

Avoid equipment or devices that sound too good to be true. Products that tout easy or effortless muscle gain and weight loss, spot reducing of thighs or waist, and super-speedy results rarely perform as the ads claim they will. The FTC has sued promoters for making exaggerated claims regarding muscle stimulators or abdominal belts that depend on electricity to "exercise" muscles.

Read the fine print. You may discover that if you want to achieve the promised gains from an exercise machine, you must also follow a specific diet—which can also trim off pounds—or do a surprising amount of exercise.

Be wary of testimonials. There's no guarantee you'll achieve the same results as satisfied customers, even if the photos aren't airbrushed. Odds are good that any celebrities pictured aren't maintaining their well-toned bodies only by using the equipment they're promoting.

Building smarter dumbbells

Dumbbells come in almost as many varieties as ice cream these days. Basic iron dumbbells are generally the cheapest option, although not necessarily the best. Sleek chrome weights look great, but can be hard to hold even when the grip is cross-hatched.

Vinyl-coated, neoprene-coated, or rubber-padded weights are more comfortable to hold and use. Some of these products are color-coded so you can easily pick out the proper weight during workouts.

A nice design in free weights uses threaded metal bars that allow you to attach weight plates at one or both ends. This versatile approach makes it easy to change weights as you gain strength. It also reduces clutter. For example, the Weider Speed Weight Adjustable Dumbbells are available in two different weight ranges, from 2.5 to 12.5 pounds and from 5 to 25 pounds. Many other systems are also available.

If your hands are arthritic, consider SoftGrip hand weights (½- to 10-pound weights) that are easy to hold. Other helpful choices include D-shaped coated weights, which are easier to grip, or wrist cuffs with pockets that hold weight bars. Choose styles that feel comfortable to you, such as gel bands or those with padded terrycloth on the inner surface. Wrist cuffs and D-shaped weights may be available only in relatively light weights, however.

You can save money on free weights by buying at a sports resale store. Check your phone book or search online. You might also score a bargain by shopping during annual or holiday sales.

Check ratings for a range of similar equipment. Check several fitness and consumer magazines. Articles aimed at people of your age and sex may be especially helpful.

Try out machines before buying. Take free tours of gyms, Y's, and community centers near your home. Ask about the weight machines they have. If one has the kind you are looking for, you might want to take advantage of a one-month or three-month membership (see "Do you need to join a gym?" on page 20). This can be a good test to see whether you would regularly use the equipment or end up hang-
Continued on page 21

Do you need to join a gym?

No one needs to join a gym to exercise regularly. Your body offers the cheapest equipment available, and spending a little money on other items can deliver great gains (see "Buying basic equipment," page 18). At home, you needn't worry about how you look to others or whether you'll have time to make it to the gym. And the money saved by not paying for a gym might be put to good use elsewhere, whether that means monthly bills or tennis lessons.

But that doesn't mean that joining a gym doesn't have its benefits. While gym memberships can be costly, spending that money may be an incentive to use the gym regularly and get your money's worth. Classes offer companionship and a safe way to learn technique (provided that the classes are geared toward your ability level). Most good gyms offer a wide range of equipment, so you can try out a variety of strength training machines and exercises. New equipment and a changing roster of exercise classes can keep you challenged and interested in working out. Often, personal trainers are available for weekly appointments or short-term overhauls of your routine. And some gyms offer a post-workout sauna, steam room, or whirlpool that can serve as a nice reward.

Before deciding whether a gym is right for you, consider your preferences and needs. Ask yourself some questions: Do you prefer to work out alone or with others? How far must you travel to the gym, and are you likely to make the trek? Do the gym's hours of operation work well for you? A home gym offers convenience (no travel time to get a workout in) and greater flexibility (you can exercise at midnight or 5 a.m. if you wish). But consider whether family interruptions might interfere with a regular workout.

If you decide to select a gym, look for the following:

A good match between your goals and the facility. Plush surroundings and a wide range of amenities cost more. Consider what you really will use—classes, trainers, or just equipment—and ignore the rest. Do, however, choose a gym that's well equipped; a variety of strength training machines and exercise classes allows you to mix up your routine and avoid boredom. And having plenty of equipment can mean no wait, or at least a shorter one, when the gym is busy. Also, be sure that the strength training machines fit you and that resistance is easy to adjust. Because most machines are made with men in mind, this is especially important for women. Take advantage of the fact that many commercial gyms will let you try their facilities for a few days or a week before making a commitment. Make sure you would feel comfortable at the gym during the hours you would normally go.

If you have significant health issues—such as disabling arthritis, a hip replacement, or a serious heart condition—a gym at a hospital or rehabilitation center may offer the best workout for you. Many of these facilities have gyms run by well-trained staff.

Well-trained staff. Expertise in teaching people to use strength training equipment and free weights is essential. Ask about staff background and training. Certification from an accredited organization, such as the American College of Sports Medicine or the American Council on Exercise, is a good sign. Ask whether staff members can perform cardiopulmonary resuscitation (CPR) if necessary. Is a defibrillator available, and do staff members know how to use it? Find out if any trainers frequently work with people of your age, level of fitness, and health status. If you regularly take medications, ask if they know how that

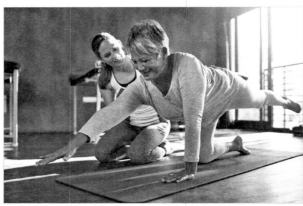

Before joining a gym, consider what amenities you need—classes or just equipment? Look for a well-trained staff who can show you how to perform exercises safely.

© PeopleImages | Getty Images

might affect your ability to work out. A friendly, helpful staff is a plus.

Cost that fits your needs. The Y, community centers, storefront gyms, and even local Boys Clubs and Girls Clubs often offer adult memberships at reasonable prices. Some health care plans offer members discounted rates at specific gyms. Working out only during off-peak hours can also cut costs in some places. In addition, some facilities let you choose to forgo certain amenities—such as a sauna, shower room, or certain classes—for a discount. Seniors can often find low-cost or free strength training classes through their local council on aging, senior center, or www.SilverSneakers.com.

A well-maintained facility. Before signing a contract, check to make sure that the gym keeps its equipment in good working order. Ask current members if machines are frequently out of order and how long it takes for broken equipment to be repaired or replaced. Also, note whether the public spaces and locker rooms appear clean and well kept.

Continued from page 19

ing clothes on it. Plus, staff members can help you learn to use it safely.

Otherwise, take your time when trying equipment at a showroom or sporting goods store to check for comfort and ease of use. Make sure you understand how to use the equipment properly. Consider the dimensions to ensure it will fit in your space. Also, do not buy equipment that cannot be adjusted to fit your body size.

Make sure it's easy to increase the resistance or add weight in increments of 5 pounds or less. Sometimes changing weights is harder than it looks, so try it out. Certain machines can be used with magnetic add-on weights in smaller amounts; ask if that's possible for the machine you're considering.

Look for good construction and safety features. Strong materials and welds and smooth action are essential. Equipment that is cheap is more likely to be flimsy and unsafe.

Double check the price. The FTC warns that "easy installment" payment plans may not include shipping and handling, tax, and set-up costs. Ask exactly what's included. And of course, shop around for the best price.

Consider customer support. Call toll-free numbers and chat with employees to get an idea of customer support. This is a good time to ask about money-back guarantees and warranties, which may be less enticing if you are responsible for paying to return an item.

Be careful when buying secondhand equipment. It is cheaper, but warranties aren't likely to apply, and usually you cannot return equipment. If you buy from a gym, the equipment is more likely to be heavy-duty. However, it's also more likely to have seen heavy use.

Personal trainers, physical therapists, and physiatrists

You can certainly follow an exercise program on your own, but exercise professionals can be helpful in certain situations, especially if you want to learn new exercises or are recovering from a health problem.

Perhaps best known are certified personal trainers. These exercise professionals offer one-on-one or small-group sessions to teach you to work out safely and maintain good form, introduce you to new equipment, and update an exercise program to keep you motivated. They also might push you to work harder than you would on your own.

If you are recovering from certain health problems, you may need to see a physical therapist instead of a personal trainer. Physical therapists help restore abilities to people with health conditions or injuries that affect muscles, joints, bones, or nerves. They create exercise plans that are safe, given a person's injury or medical condition, and they help each client perform the exercise correctly. A physical therapist may specialize in cardiopulmonary rehabilitation, orthopedics, sports medicine, geriatrics, or another area.

Physiatrists are medical doctors who specialize in physical medicine and rehabilitation. They treat people who face significant pain, muscle or bone injuries, nerve damage, or conditions such as stroke, hip fracture, or spinal cord injuries that require rehabilitation. Some have specialties, such as pediatrics, geriatrics, musculoskeletal medicine, or neurological injuries. While physiatrists may tell you what exercises and movements not to do, they generally leave it up to physical therapists to design exercise programs for their patients.

Insurance coverage varies; in some cases, your

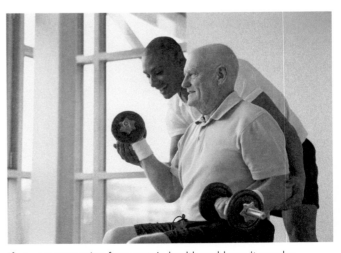

If you are recovering from certain health problems, it may be advisable to work with a physical therapist at first. He or she will create an exercise plan that's safe for you, given your condition.

insurance may pay for a specific number of sessions with a physical therapist or physiatrist if you are diagnosed with a condition that the company believes warrants the use of such services. Check with your insurance provider to learn more.

Choosing wisely

When selecting an exercise professional, always ask about credentials and experience. Find out how often the person works with people of your age, abilities, and overall health.

In some states, just about anyone can claim to be a personal trainer. Look for someone with certification from an accredited organization such as the American College of Sports Medicine (ACSM) or the American Council on Exercise (ACE). You may be able to locate a personal trainer through recommendations from friends or by calling local gyms, Y's, and community or senior centers. Or check with the ACSM or ACE (see "Resources," page 51).

Physical therapists must complete training and pass a national exam given by the Federation of State Boards of Physical Therapy. They should be licensed by the state in which they practice. Those who complete advanced training in specialized areas must take additional exams to become board-certified specialists.

Physiatrists must complete full medical training and an accredited residency program in their field. Some specialize in specific areas, so it's worth checking beforehand. All must pass written and oral exams given by the American Board of Physical Medicine and Rehabilitation.

If you have significant health problems or disabilities, you can benefit from consulting with a professional who understands your condition before you launch a program of strength or power training. Your primary care physician may be able to refer you to the appropriate person, or you can call rehabilitation centers and hospitals in your area to see if they offer helpful exercise programs for people in your situation. ♥

Safety first

When you were younger, you probably never thought twice about starting an exercise program. You just went to the gym and signed up. As you age, however, it's wise to consult with your doctor or physical therapist before starting a program of strength or power training. He or she can tell you whether you need to start slowly or take any precautions, such as avoiding certain exercises. It is especially important that you talk to your doctor if you have not been active recently, or if you have any injuries or a chronic or unstable health condition, such as any of these:

- heart disease (or multiple risk factors for it)
- a respiratory ailment such as asthma
- high blood pressure
- joint or bone disease
- a neurologic illness
- diabetes.

Some conditions, such as unstable angina or an abdominal aortic aneurysm (a weak spot in the wall of the body's main artery) can make strength or power training unsafe. Other problems—for example, a joint injury or cataract treatment—may make it unsafe

temporarily; in that case, wait until your doctor gives you the go-ahead.

You may also want to use a helpful tool developed by the Canadian Society for Exercise Physiology. Called the Get Active Questionnaire, this series of questions can help you determine whether you should talk to your doctor before embarking on, or ramping up, any exercise program. You can find it online at www.health. harvard.edu/GAQ. The form covers people of all ages.

Generally speaking, anyone who is healthy or has a well-controlled health problem, such as high blood pressure or diabetes, can safely do strength and power training. That includes frail older people. But some people will need more supervision or must observe more restrictions than others. Your doctor is the best person to advise you.

Questions for your doctor

If you do want or need to speak to a doctor, bring, fax, or email descriptions of the exercises in this report that you plan to do, and ask if you can safely undertake them. Your doctor may feel your selections are fine or might wish to modify certain moves or suggest substitutions. Here are four good questions to ask:

1 Would any of my health conditions be adversely affected by strength or power training or other types of exercise? (For example, people with poorly controlled high blood pressure generally should avoid isometric exercises, such as the back extension, page 39, which can raise blood pressure considerably.)

2 Will my medications affect exercise in any way or vice versa? (People taking insulin or medicine to lower blood sugar may need to adjust the dose when they exercise, for example.)

3 Should I have any limits on the types or intensity of exercises I do? (For example, some people who have had a hip replacement may be told to avoid bringing their knees to their chests.)

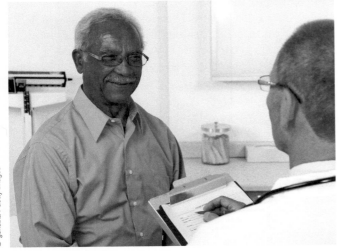

Generally speaking, anyone who is healthy or has a well-controlled health problem, such as high blood pressure or diabetes, can safely do strength and power training. But check with your doctor first.

4 Do I need supervision while I exercise? (See "Do you need supervision?" below right.)

If necessary, your doctor can refer you to a physiatrist, a physical therapist, or another specialist for evaluation (see "Personal trainers, physical therapists, and physiatrists," page 21).

When you may need to stop exercising

The National Institute on Aging notes that there are also specific reasons to hold off temporarily on exercise until a doctor advises you that it's safe to resume. These are not specific to strength training; you should not do aerobic exercise, either, if you have any of the following:

- a hernia
- sores on feet or ankles that aren't healing
- hot, swollen joints
- difficulty walking, or lasting pain, after a fall
- blood clots
- a detached or bleeding retina, cataract surgery or a lens implant, or laser eye surgery
- a fever (it is usually safe to start exercising again at lighter intensity once the fever has subsided and you feel better)
- an irregular, fast, or fluttery heartbeat.

In addition, there are a number of warning signs that should prompt a call to your doctor (see "Warning signs," page 25).

Tips for avoiding injury

Strength training is quite safe for most people as long as they take certain precautions. In addition to getting advice from your doctor or other health professional, it's wise to follow these guidelines for avoiding injury:

- Always warm up and cool down properly (see "Why should I warm up and cool down?" on page 29).
- Use proper form to avoid injuries and maximize gains. It's easiest to learn good form through a class or one-on-one sessions with a well-trained exercise professional. If that's not possible, exercise in front of a mirror so you can check your form (see "What is good form?" on page 28).
- Breathe out when you are lifting or pushing; breathe in as you slowly release the load or weight. Never hold your breath while straining. This action, called the Valsalva maneuver, can raise your blood pressure considerably and can be risky for people with cardiovascular disease. Counting out loud as you lift will prevent you from holding your breath.
- Lift or push and release weights slowly and smoothly, without jerking. Jerky movements can lead to spraining or straining a muscle, tendon, or ligament.
- Don't lock your joints; always leave a slight bend in your knees and elbows when straightening out your legs and arms. Hyperextended joints can strain ligaments around the joint.
- Bend at the hips, not at the waist, and keep your back straight and abdominal muscles contracted in order to protect your back muscles.
- Work evenly at the pace specified in each exercise.

Do you need supervision?

Nearly everyone can exercise, and certainly the vast majority of us should. But for some people it's safest to do so with good supervision. This simple test can help you determine whether you can safely exercise without supervision at home or at a gym, or whether it would be best to work with qualified exercise professionals at a gym, senior center, rehabilitation center, or hospital (see "Personal trainers, physical therapists, and physiatrists," page 21). Classes taught by well-trained exercise professionals could also be an option, if individual sessions aren't possible.

The test focuses on your levels of strength and balance. Answer each question with a **"yes"** or **"no."**

Questions	YES	NO
Can you do one chair stand (page 32) without using your arms to assist you?		
Can you walk up and down a flight of 10 stairs without using the handrail to balance yourself?		
Can you stand unsupported on one foot for five seconds?		
Can you perform each of these exercises without discomfort?		

If you answered "no" to any of these questions, you can certainly still exercise, but you should do so in a supervised environment.

Warning signs

These warning signs pertain to any kind of exercise—strength and power training and aerobic exercise alike.

Signs of an emergency

If you experience any of these symptoms during or after exercise, call 911 or see a doctor immediately:

- chest pain, pressure, heaviness, or tightness
- faintness or loss of consciousness
- significant or persistent shortness of breath or dizziness.

Ask your doctor whether any other warning signs specific to your health history warrant a call.

Signs that you should call your doctor for advice

Persistent or intense muscle pain that starts during a session or right afterward, or muscle soreness that persists more than one to two weeks, merits a call to your doctor for advice. (This is in contrast to the normal muscle soreness that starts 12 to 48 hours after an exercise session and gradually abates.)

You should also call your doctor if the routine you've been doing for a while without discomfort starts to cause you pain.

Control is very important. Counting off the tempo aloud helps you stay in control, which enhances gains and helps you avoid injuries. It also ensures that you're breathing, rather than holding your breath.

- When moving your arms or legs, stick with a range that feels comfortable. These exercises should not cause pain while you are doing them. Over time, gradually extend your range of motion through exercise and stretching.
- Don't overexert yourself. Listen to your body and cut back if you aren't able to finish a series of exercises or an exercise session, can't talk while exercising, feel faint after a session, feel tired during the day, or suffer joint aches and pains after a session.
- Build up slowly over time. Don't be so eager to see results that you risk hurting yourself by exercising too long or choosing too much weight. Remember that it's important to rest muscles for at least 48 hours between sessions.
- If you've been sick, give yourself one or two days off after recovering. If you were ill for a while, you may need to use lighter weights or less resistance when you first resume exercising.
- Slow down if the temperature where you exercise is higher than 70° F. When it tops 80° F, try to exercise only during the coolest part of the day. Dress in loose, light clothes. Headache, dizziness, nausea, fainting, cramps, or palpitations are signs of overheating.
- Drink plenty of water throughout the day and whenever you exercise in order to prevent headaches and fatigue. As people age, their sense of thirst declines, so it's particularly important for older adults to drink lots of water when they exercise (and during the day, as well)—even if they don't feel thirsty.
- Soreness is normal for a day or two after strength or power training sessions, especially when you first start to work out. But you shouldn't feel overly tired or have sore joints or specific muscle injuries.
- If you injure yourself, remember RICE (rest, ice, compression, and elevation). Rest the injured muscle. Ice it for 20 to 30 minutes every two to three hours during the first two or three days. Apply compression with an elastic bandage whenever you're out of bed until the swelling resolves. Elevate the injured area while resting or icing. Call your doctor for advice and information about managing pain or swelling. Wait until the injury heals before doing strength training on that muscle again, and start with a lower weight. ▼

Designing your program

Before you lift even the lightest weight, you need to answer certain questions. How often should you do strength training? How about power training? What are "reps" and "sets," and how many should you do? How much weight or resistance should you use? How much time should you spend doing your warm-up, cool-down, rest, and stretches? This chapter covers these issues and more. You will also learn what a well-rounded exercise program should include in addition to strength training (see "Current exercise recommendations," page 29).

After you've read this information, proceed to the weekly workout planner (page 27), where you can write up a schedule for the program you plan to follow each week.

Frequently asked questions

The answers to the following questions provide crucial information about strength training.

How often should I do strength training?

According to the most recent Physical Activity Guidelines for Americans, issued by the U.S. Department of Health and Human Services, adults should perform a complete strength training routine two or three times a week. (Of course, once a week is better than not at all, if that's the most you can manage.) The fastest gains are made in the first four to eight weeks; after that, expect progress to slow somewhat.

How often should I do power training?

The Physical Activity Guidelines for Americans do not address power training, but the American College of Sports Medicine has been advocating it for 10 years. Based on research, it recommends doing power training two or three times a week along with strength training. You can easily do that with the workouts in this report.

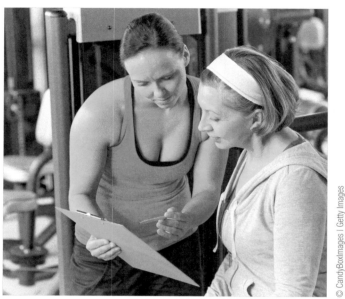

A trainer can help you draw up an exercise program that includes aerobic and strength training plus balance exercises, if you need them. Be sure to allow 48 hours between strength sessions.

© CandyBoxImages | Getty Images

How much rest do my muscles need?

Always allow at least 48 hours for muscles to recover between strength training sessions. So, if you do a full-body strength workout on Monday, wait until at least Wednesday to repeat it.

Some people prefer to break their strength training program into two components: upper body and lower body. In that case, you can perform upper-body exercises one day and lower-body exercises the next. Just make sure you work different groups of muscles on successive days, so your muscles can rest properly. And remember, you'll need to schedule at least two to three upper-body workouts and two to three lower-body workouts a week.

What are "reps" and "sets"?

Most strength training routines call for lifting and lowering a weight eight to 12 times, or repetitions ("reps"). That makes up one set. Typically, a complete

Continued on page 28

Weekly workout planner

Week: _____ / _____ / _____ to _____ / _____ / _____

SUNDAY	MONDAY	TUESDAY	WEDNESDAY	THURSDAY	FRIDAY	SATURDAY
Time _____ Activity _____ Duration _____ ☐ Done	Time _____ Activity _____ Duration _____ ☐ Done	Time _____ Activity _____ Duration _____ ☐ Done	Time _____ Activity _____ Duration _____ ☐ Done	Time _____ Activity _____ Duration _____ ☐ Done	Time _____ Activity _____ Duration _____ ☐ Done	Time _____ Activity _____ Duration _____ ☐ Done
Time _____ Activity _____ Duration _____ ☐ Done	Time _____ Activity _____ Duration _____ ☐ Done	Time _____ Activity _____ Duration _____ ☐ Done	Time _____ Activity _____ Duration _____ ☐ Done	Time _____ Activity _____ Duration _____ ☐ Done	Time _____ Activity _____ Duration _____ ☐ Done	Time _____ Activity _____ Duration _____ ☐ Done
Time _____ Activity _____ Duration _____ ☐ Done	Time _____ Activity _____ Duration _____ ☐ Done	Time _____ Activity _____ Duration _____ ☐ Done	Time _____ Activity _____ Duration _____ ☐ Done	Time _____ Activity _____ Duration _____ ☐ Done	Time _____ Activity _____ Duration _____ ☐ Done	Time _____ Activity _____ Duration _____ ☐ Done
Notes _____ _____ _____ _____	Notes _____ _____ _____ _____	Notes _____ _____ _____ _____	Notes _____ _____ _____ _____	Notes _____ _____ _____ _____	Notes _____ _____ _____ _____	Notes _____ _____ _____ _____

Continued from page 26

workout includes two to three sets of approximately eight to 12 exercises that, combined, exercise all the major muscle groups.

For power training, you will do fewer reps—six to 10—but at a faster pace.

What is good form?

Before you attempt a specific exercise, it's essential to learn the proper form, or technique, for the equipment and exercise you've chosen. Good form means aligning your head, shoulders, spine, hips, knees, and ankles correctly for each move, maintaining balance, and moving smoothly through the exercise. Hunching over, thrusting your hips forward, turning your knees in, or performing jerky motions are examples of poor form. Focus on slow, smooth lifts and descents while isolating a muscle group. You isolate, or target, muscle groups by holding your body in a specific position while you contract or release certain muscles. Keep joints slightly bent rather than locked when you're extending the muscles. By observing good form, you strengthen that targeted muscle group and avoid unnecessary strain on other muscles. In contrast, poor form can cause injuries and—at best—slow gains. (See "Tips for avoiding injury," page 24.)

Strength training machines can help position you properly. But you still need to learn to adjust each machine to your body and use it correctly. If you're using free weights for resistance, good form is even more essential. Often, it helps to run through exercises the first few times without weights or with very little weight. A class or exercise professional can be instrumental in teaching good form. Videos and books can help, too.

It's also a good idea to exercise in front of a mirror, at least initially. This lets you observe your body position and correct sloppy form.

How much weight or resistance should I use?

As you are learning a new exercise, use a very light weight or none at all so you can concentrate on good form. Once you are comfortable performing an exercise, choose a weight that allows you to do only eight to 12 repetitions. The last one or two reps should be difficult. If you can't lift the weight at least eight times, use a lighter weight. You can adjust the amount of weight you are lifting for subsequent sets based on how you feel.

If you exercise regularly, your muscles will gradually adapt to the weight you are using so you can do more reps. When you can comfortably perform 12 reps without completely tiring the muscle, it's time to increase the amount of weight. Muscles grow stronger only if you keep adding weight.

How fast should I lift the weights?

The speed, or tempo, at which you perform the exercises will vary depending upon the type of exercise you are doing. Strength training exercises should be done at a seven-second tempo. That means three seconds to lift the weight (while exhaling), a one-second pause, and three seconds to lower it (while inhaling). For power training, you'll pick up the pace. You will do the lifting as quickly as possible while maintaining good form. You will hold at the top of the move for one second. Then you will take three seconds to lower.

How many sets should I do?

Strength training focuses on tiring the muscles that are being worked. When you are beginning a program, start with two sets of eight repetitions and work

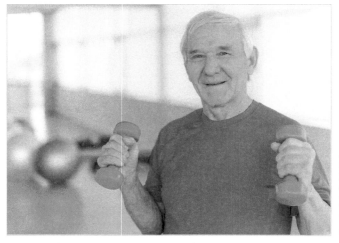

Focus on slow, smooth motions when lifting weights, and be especially careful to control the descent. By observing good form, you strengthen the targeted muscles and help avoid injuries.

up from there; if you cannot perform eight repetitions initially, do as many as you can (or reduce the weight or do only one set). When you can comfortably do two to three sets of 12 repetitions, increase the weight.

How long should I rest between sets?

Resting for a minute or two between sets nets the best strength gains. If you don't rest at all, your muscles will be too tired to lift with good form. A slightly longer rest period after power training sets may be desirable. Listen to your body and take more rest time whenever you need it.

Why should I warm up and cool down?

Warming up pumps nutrient-rich, oxygenated blood to your muscles as it raises your heart rate and breathing to prepare for exercise. Cooling down slows breathing and heartbeat, gradually routing blood back into its normal circulatory patterns. This helps prevent a sudden drop in blood pressure that causes dizziness, especially if you bend over or straighten up quickly (a reaction called postural hypotension).

You should always begin your exercise session by warming up for five to 10 minutes, and end by cooling down for another five to 10 minutes. Excellent ways to warm up include marching in place and gently swinging your arms, walking on a treadmill, pedaling an exercise bike, or mimicking an exercise without holding any weights. Start slowly, and gradually increase your pace. (Stretching is no longer recommended as a warm-up, unless it's a "dynamic" stretch that involves movement; to see a short routine, go to www.health.harvard.edu/dynamic-stretches.)

To cool down, gradually slow your movements or walk slowly until your heart rate and breathing are close to normal. Then do some stretching.

Why—and when—should I stretch?

Stretching can help you work kinks out of a stiff neck, ease back pain, and grasp a zipper that's been out of reach for years. Daily stretching gives you a greater range of motion and improves balance, too. The best time to stretch is not at the beginning of a workout, but rather at the end of the session, when your mus-

A strong exercise routine

For your exercise routine, aim for the following:

- at least 150 minutes of moderate aerobic activity, or 75 minutes of vigorous activity, or an equivalent mix per week (even a minute or two of activity counts)

- two to three sessions per week of strength training that exercises the major muscle groups of the legs, trunk, and arms and shoulders—or four to six weekly sessions if you plan to exercise only upper-body muscles on one day and lower-body muscles on the following day

- power training as part of your strength routine; the Physical Activity Guidelines for Americans do not yet include power training, but research supports including this element

- balance exercises, either as part of your strength training routine or separately

- stretching exercises during the cool-down portion of each exercise session.

cles are warm and pliable (see "Balancing and stretching exercises," page 40).

Yoga, tai chi, and Pilates, which can be tailored to differing abilities and health concerns, combine stretching with relaxation. Studies show these activities enhance balance, lower blood pressure, and relieve stress, as well as improve flexibility.

Current exercise recommendations

Strength training is only one piece of the exercise puzzle, of course. It's wise to keep the bigger picture in mind. A well-rounded program also includes aerobic activity, flexibility exercises, and balance exercises (see "A strong exercise routine," above). And most of the research shows that combined programs, especially those including both aerobic exercise and strength training, provide greater benefits than doing either solo.

Aerobic activity (also called cardiovascular or endurance exercise), such as walking or swimming, speeds heart rate and breathing for sustained periods. According to the Physical Activity Guidelines for Americans, most adults should aim for at least 150 minutes of moderate aerobic activity per week or 75 minutes of vigorous activity—or an equiva-

There are various ways to determine how hard you are exercising. But this one, known informally as the "talk test," is simple and intuitive: if you can sing and do the activity, it is low intensity; if you can carry on a conversation but not sing, it is moderate intensity; and if you can speak only a few words at a time, it is vigorous or high intensity.

lent mix of the two. (Ten minutes of vigorous activity equals roughly 20 minutes of moderate activity.) Raising your weekly goal to five hours of moderate activity or two-and-a-half hours of vigorous activity nets additional health benefits and may be helpful if one of your goals is weight loss. Spread your aerobic exercise across the week, so that you are exercising at least three days a week. Even a few minutes of activity count.

According to many exercise guidelines, running is an example of "vigorous" aerobic exercise. "Moderate" exercise might be walking at 3.5 mph. The truth is, though, your level of fitness dictates whether an activity is light, moderate, or vigorous. If you are rarely active, a less-than-brisk walk might qualify as moderate—or even vigorous. (See "How hard are you exercising?" above for a simple way to gauge your level of exertion.) Many experts also offer the following rule of thumb for aerobic exercise: If you can talk easily while

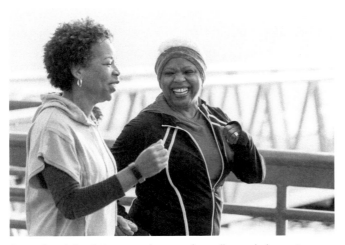

Strength training is just one element of a well-rounded exercise plan. Aerobic exercise, such as walking or running, is also essential. Aim for at least 150 minutes of aerobic exercise per week.

performing your routine, exercise harder. If you can't carry on a conversation at all, back off.

Flexibility exercises, or stretches, may expand your range of motion, keep muscles more limber, improve posture and balance, and help prevent falls. You receive the most benefits from stretches when your muscles are warm and pliable, so it's best to perform them as part of your cool-down following a workout. Or, if you prefer, you can stretch after a five- to 10-minute warm-up, during which you might walk or dance to some songs on the radio. Consider activities such as yoga or tai chi, which help with balance as well as flexibility. The American College of Sports Medicine recommends that older adults do flexibility exercises on the same days they do aerobic or strength activities, or at least twice a week.

Because regularly performing balance exercises can help protect against falls, it's wise to include these kinds of exercises in your routine. Here, you may be happy to note that your strength training routine can do double duty. Several of the strength training exercises described in this report also improve balance, particularly standing calf raises (page 32), chair stands (page 32), hip extensions (page 33), and side leg raises (page 38). We've also included two separate balance exercises that are simple to perform (see "Balancing," page 40).

A good exercise program builds slowly and safely on your current level of fitness. If you're a beginner, don't despair. Work up to these goals gradually. You'll find that some of these activities overlap nicely. For example, strength training has aerobic benefits if it raises your heart rate for sustained periods of time. You needn't follow a formula to know exactly how much faster than usual your heart should be beating— just pay attention to body signals that suggest you are exercising moderately (see "How hard are you exercising?" above left). And remember to stretch as part of your cool-down.

Your workout calendar

With all of this information, you are now ready to design your program. Start by making copies of the weekly workout planner on page 27. Then fill in the dates of the coming week on one page. Schedule days and times for your strength training. Add in aerobic activities and flexibility exercises, too. When you do a workout, check it off. If you miss a workout, jot down the reason. This can help you see when it's easiest to incorporate exercise into your schedule and where roadblocks tend to crop up. At the end of the week, review the calendar to see whether you need to make any adjustments in the timing of your workouts.

This report lays out two different strength training workouts. Which one is the best match for you? If you aren't usually active at all, focus on the strength training program in Workout I and gradually add aerobic activities when you can. Even a few minutes a day will help, especially if you try to do a bit more week by week. Although it seems counterintuitive to start with strength training, it is a good way to build up muscles that are too weak for walking and other aerobic activities. If you are in good shape, you may wish to use the strength training program in Workout II.

After you have completed one of these programs for 12 to 16 weeks, see the Special Section of this report ("Strength training over a lifetime," page 44) to find out how to maintain your strength gains and keep your strength training routine fun and challenging. No matter which program you start with, get a baseline of your current abilities by completing the first column of the "Progress chart" on page 45. Then chart the changes month by month. This will allow you to see and celebrate all the improvements you make. ◆

Workout I: A strong beginning

Building the strength and power you need for daily tasks and recreation is one major goal of these exercises, which were designed with beginners in mind. By focusing on muscles you actually use to walk up stairs, rise from a chair, or lift laundry or groceries, these exercises can help you maintain these abilities as you get older or even regain them if you've already lost them. This is known as specificity—that is, choosing activities that target the specific muscles and moves needed for the tasks of daily life (or a particular sport) rather than just building up muscles in gen-

eral. In addition, the power moves in this workout can help you boost your ability to bring muscle force to bear quickly. That could make the difference between catching yourself after a misstep or falling.

Because this program has just nine exercises, it's easier and less intimidating than many other strength training regimens. Make it your goal to complete 12 to 16 weeks of Workout I, performing these exercises two to three times a week. If you do, you will notice many changes for the better. As you grow stronger, activities of all sorts will become easier. Simple tasks

Workout I

1 Standing calf raise

Exercises the calf muscles

Stand with your feet flat on the floor. Hold on to the back of your chair for balance. Raise yourself up on the balls of your feet, as high as possible. Hold briefly, then lower yourself. Do eight to 12 repetitions. Rest and repeat the set.

Harder variation: Once your balance and strength improve, do one-leg calf raises. Tuck one foot behind the other calf before rising on the ball of your foot; do sets for each leg. Or try doing calf raises without holding on to a chair.

Power move: Rise up on the balls of your feet quickly. Hold briefly. Lower yourself at a normal pace. Do six to 10 repetitions.

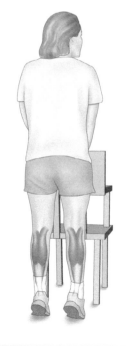

2 Chair stand

Exercises the muscles of the abdomen, hips, front thighs, and buttocks

Place a small pillow at the back of your chair and position the chair so that the back of it is resting against a wall. Sit at the front of the chair, knees bent, feet flat on the floor and slightly apart. Lean back on the pillow in a half-reclining position with your arms crossed and your hands on your shoulders. While keeping your back and shoulders straight, raise your upper body forward until you are sitting upright. Stand up slowly, using your hands as little as possible. Slowly sit back down. Do eight to 12 repetitions. Rest and repeat the set.

Easier variation: Use your hands to help you stand up.

Power move: Rise from the chair quickly. Sit down again at a normal pace. Do six to 10 repetitions.

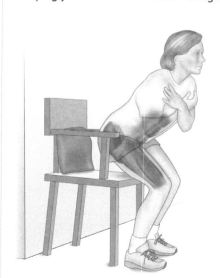

such as rising from a chair or going up stairs will no longer be a challenge. Sports may seem more enjoyable or simply become possible again. You may lose some weight or perhaps just feel as if you've lost some, because your waistband will loosen as your abdominal muscles firm up. Even better are the changes you cannot see that put you on the road toward a healthier heart and bones and a lower risk of diabetes.

What you need. A sturdy chair (preferably with armrests), a small pillow, athletic shoes with non-skid soles, an exercise mat, and appropriate weights (see "Buying basic equipment," page 18) are all that you need. When choosing ankle weights and dumbbells, find weights that are challenging for you, even if they're light. Remember, you should increase the amount of weight you use whenever an exercise starts to feel easy (usually about every week or two).

Performing the exercises

Before beginning the workout, complete a five- to 10-minute warm-up, such as marching in place. As you perform each of these exercises, breathe out when you are lifting or pushing, and breathe in as you release the muscle. Rest for one to two minutes between sets, and aim to complete two to three sets of each exercise. Don't forget to cool down at the end of the session.

Start by doing the exercises without the power option for about four weeks. After the first month or so, try making the last set of each exercise the one with the power move. For variety, you could also do your power set first. When you do power sets, you'll lift as fast as possible. Pause for a moment at the top of the move, then slowly lower for about three seconds.

3 Stair climbing

Exercises the muscles of the front thighs and buttocks

Holding on to the handrail for balance if necessary, walk up and down a flight of at least 10 stairs at a pace that feels comfortable. Pause at the top only if you need to do so. Rest when you reach the bottom. Repeat four times.

Power move: If your balance is good, go up the stairs as briskly as you can and come back down at your normal pace. Repeat twice for a total of three times.

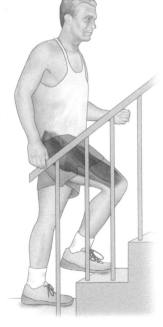

4 Hip extension

Exercises the muscles of the buttocks and back thighs

While wearing ankle weights, stand 12 inches behind a sturdy chair. Holding on to the back of the chair for balance, bend your trunk forward 45°. Slowly raise your right leg straight out behind you. Lift it as high as possible without bending your knee. Pause. Slowly lower the leg. Do eight to 12 repetitions. Repeat with your left leg. Rest and repeat the sets.

Easier variation: Do this move without the ankle weights.

Power move: Lift your leg quickly. Hold briefly. Lower your leg at a normal pace. Do six to 10 repetitions.

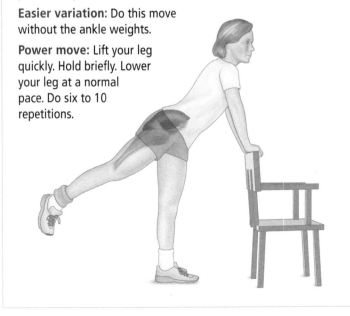

5 Seated bridge

Exercises the muscles of the back thighs, back, and buttocks

Sit slightly forward in a chair with your hands on the armrests. Your feet should be flat on the floor and slightly apart, and your upper body should be upright (don't lean forward). Using your arms for balance only, slowly raise your buttocks off the chair until you are nearly standing, with your knees bent. Pause. Slowly sit back down. Do eight to 12 repetitions. Rest and repeat the set.

Power move: Rise out of the chair quickly. Hold briefly. Lower yourself at a normal pace. Do six to 10 repetitions.

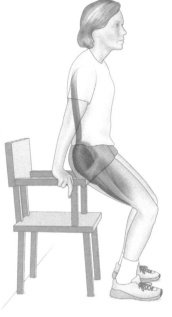

6 Biceps curl

Exercises the front upper arm muscles

Sit in a chair. Hold weights down at your sides with your palms inward. Slowly bend one elbow, lifting the weight toward your upper chest. As you lift, keep your elbow close to your side and rotate your palm so it faces your shoulder. Pause. Slowly lower your arm, rotating it back again so you finish with your palm facing your thighs. Do eight to 12 repetitions. Repeat with your other arm. Rest and repeat the set.

Power move: Lift the weight quickly. Hold briefly. Lower the weight at a normal pace. Do six to 10 repetitions.

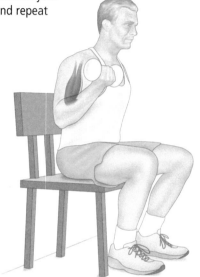

7 Triceps dip

Exercises the muscles of the back upper arms, chest, and shoulders

Put a chair with armrests up against a wall. Sit in the chair and put your feet together flat on the floor. Lean forward a bit while keeping your shoulders and back straight. Bend your elbows and place your hands on the armrests of the chair, so they are in line with your torso. Pressing downward on your hands, try to lift yourself up a few inches by straightening out your arms. Raise your upper body and thighs, but keep your feet in contact with the floor. Pause. Slowly release until you're sitting back down again. Do eight to 12 repetitions. Rest and repeat the set.

If you don't have a chair with armrests, sit on the stairs. Put your palms down on the stair above the one you are seated on. Press downward on the heels of your hands, lifting your body a few inches as you straighten your arms. Pause. Slowly release your body until you are sitting back down again. Do eight to 12 repetitions. Rest and repeat the set.

Power move: Lift your body quickly. Hold briefly. Lower yourself at a normal pace. Do six to 10 repetitions.

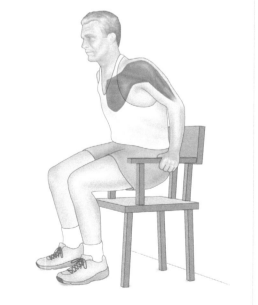

8 Curl-up*

Exercises the central abdominal muscles

Lie on your back on a mat. Put your hands beneath the small of your back and bend both knees to help stabilize your spine. Slowly raise your head and shoulders just a few inches off the floor. Pause. Slowly lower your head and shoulders. Do eight to 12 repetitions. Rest and repeat the set.

Power move: Lift your head and shoulders quickly off the floor. Hold briefly. Lower yourself at a normal pace. Do six to 10 repetitions.

If you have osteoporosis, talk to your doctor before trying this exercise. He or she may recommend that you avoid it.

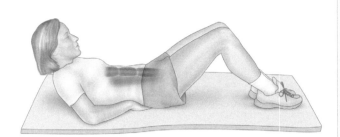

9 Standing side bridge

Exercises the lower back, sides, and abdomen

Stand next to a wall, so the wall is on your right. Position yourself about two to three feet from the wall. Place your left foot directly in front of your right, and bend your right arm at your elbow. Lean your forearm against the wall so you are tilted toward it at about a 15° angle. Keep your body and spine in a straight line. **(A)** Hold that position for 30 seconds.

Now pivot on your toes, turning so you are facing the wall. Your feet should be side-by-side. Lean both forearms against the wall. Again, keep your spine straight; don't bend the torso. **(B)** Hold for 30 seconds.

Finally, pivot on your toes again so the wall is now on your left side. Your right foot should now be in front of your left, and you should lean against the wall on your left forearm. **(C)** Hold for 30 seconds. That's one set. Rest, and repeat the whole sequence for another set. (While most exercises in this workout are performed eight to 12 times in a set, this exercise is only done once per set.)

Try to move from one position to the next as fluidly as possible, maintaining your spine in a straight line. Once you are comfortable with this exercise, increase the amount of time you hold each position by about 15-second increments, working up to two minutes at each position. ▼

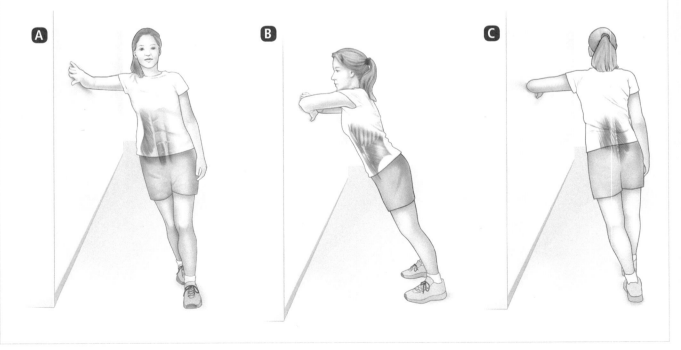

Workout II: Stepping it up a notch

If you're reasonably active or have completed at least 12 to 16 weeks of Workout I, you may want more of a challenge. Workout II focuses on the same basic muscle groups, but offers some new exercises plus variations on a few exercises from Workout I.

If you're not ready to move on to Workout II after 12 to 16 weeks of doing Workout I, you can also ease into it. Try stepping up the program in Workout I by adding weight, repetitions (up to a maximum of 12), or sets (up to a maximum of four; see "Stepping up the pace," page 46). You'll see even more improvement, though, if you also gradually add a few of the exercises from Workout II to your previous routine. Recommended additions are the reverse fly, dumbbell squat,

Workout II

1 Reverse fly

Exercises the muscles of the shoulders and upper back

Sit in a chair holding weights about 12 inches in front of your chest. Your elbows should be up and slightly bent, and palms should be facing each other (as if your arms are wrapped around a large beach ball). Lean forward at a slight angle in the chair, bending from your hips and keeping your back straight. Now, pull the weights apart while trying to bring your shoulder blades as close together as possible. Let the movement pull your elbows back as far as possible. Pause. Return to starting position. Do eight to 12 repetitions. Rest and repeat the set.

Power move: Pull the weights back quickly. Hold briefly. Bring arms back together at a normal pace. Do six to 10 repetitions.

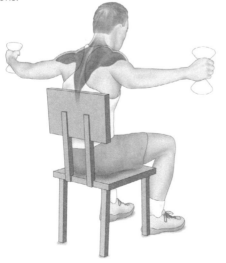

2 Overhead press

Exercises the muscles of the shoulders, upper back, and back upper arms

Stand with your feet slightly apart. Hold a dumbbell in each hand at shoulder height (your elbows should be bent, and the weights should be by your shoulders). Hold the weights so your palms are facing forward. Slowly press the weights straight up until your arms are fully extended. Pause. Slowly lower the dumbbells to shoulder level. Do eight to 12 repetitions. Rest and repeat the set.

Power move: Lift the weights quickly. Hold briefly. Lower your arms at a normal pace. Do six to 10 repetitions.

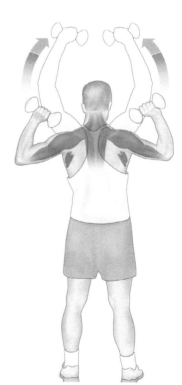

side leg raise, and back extension. Tacking on just one of these new exercises per week—or one every few weeks—should help you ease into Workout II.

After about four weeks of doing Workout II, you can add on the power moves for even greater benefits. Continue to do the power moves described in Workout I as well. If just one set seems too easy, try two or three. Or, if you prefer, turn up the power even more by wearing a weighted vest (see "How to use a weighted vest," page 46). You must keep challenging yourself as the routine becomes easier if you wish to continue to reap gains.

Perform this routine two to three times a week.

Make it your goal to complete 12 to 16 weeks of Workout II. Then, if you like, try some new exercises (see "Moving onward: Switching up your routine," page 49).

Performing the exercises

Do two or three sets of each of these exercises. Remember to breathe as you exercise, because holding your breath can raise your blood pressure dangerously high. Breathe out when you're lifting or pushing, and breathe in as you relax the muscle. Don't forget to rest for one minute between sets for the best strength training gains.

3 Triceps extension

Exercises the back upper arm muscles

Begin by standing with your feet slightly apart, holding weights with your palms facing behind you. Lift the weights straight up. As you lift, you'll be raising your elbows up and bending them at about a 90° angle. Your shoulders should not hunch up, and your elbows should not be any higher than your shoulders. If you feel any shoulder pain, lower your arms slightly. This is the starting position. While keeping your elbows at the same level, slowly raise your forearms out to your sides so your arms are outstretched. Pause. Slowly return to the starting position. Do eight to 12 repetitions. Rest and repeat the set.

Another option: If this exercise causes you any shoulder pain, try the triceps dip (page 34) in Workout I.

Power move: Straighten your arms quickly. Hold briefly. Bend your arms at a normal pace. Do six to 10 repetitions.

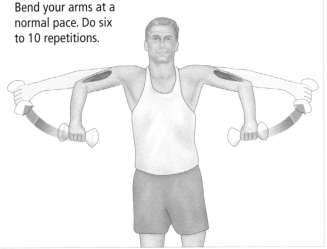

4 Double biceps curl

Exercises the front upper arm muscles

Stand or sit holding dumbbells down at your sides with your palms facing inward. Slowly bend both elbows, lifting the weights toward your upper chest. Keep your elbows close to your sides. As you lift, rotate your palms so they face your shoulders. Pause. Slowly lower your arms to the starting position. Do eight to 12 repetitions. Rest and repeat the set.

Power move: Lift the weights quickly. Hold briefly. Lower the weights at a normal pace. Do six to 10 repetitions.

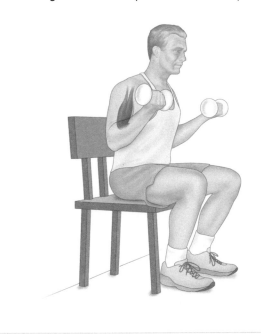

5 Dumbbell squat

Exercises the muscles of the buttocks and front thighs

Stand with your feet apart. Hold a weight in each hand with your arms at your sides and palms facing inward. Slowly

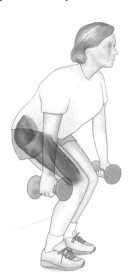

bend your hips and knees, leaning forward no more than 45° and lowering your buttocks down and back about eight inches. Don't round or excessively arch your back as you do this. Pause. Slowly rise to an upright position. Do eight to 12 repetitions. Rest and repeat the set.

Easier variation: Do this move without holding weights.

Power move: Lower yourself at a normal pace. Hold briefly. Stand up quickly. Do six to 10 repetitions.

6 Side leg raise

Exercises the muscles of the hips and sides of thighs

Wearing an ankle weight, stand behind a sturdy chair with

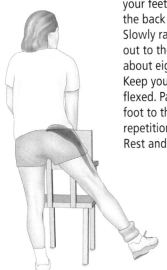

your feet together. Hold on to the back of the chair for balance. Slowly raise your right leg straight out to the side until your foot is about eight inches off the floor. Keep your knee straight and foot flexed. Pause. Slowly lower your foot to the floor. Do eight to 12 repetitions. Repeat with left leg. Rest and repeat the set.

Easier variation: Do this move without the ankle weight.

Power move: Lift your leg quickly. Hold briefly. Lower your leg at a normal pace. Do six to 10 repetitions.

7 Bridge

Exercises the muscles of the back, back thighs, and buttocks

Lie on your back on a mat with your knees bent and your feet flat on the floor. Put your hands next to your hips with palms flat on the floor. Keep your back straight as you lift your buttocks as high as you can off the mat, using your hands for balance only. Pause. Lower your buttocks without touching the mat, then lift again. Do eight to 12 repetitions. Rest and repeat the set.

Power move: Lift your buttocks quickly. Hold briefly. Lower your buttocks at a normal pace. Do six to 10 repetitions.

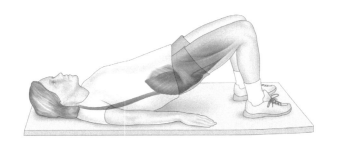

8 Advanced curl-up*

Exercises the abdominal muscles

Lie on your back on a mat. Put your hands beneath the small of your back and bend both knees to help stabilize your spine. While contracting your abdominal muscles so your navel is pulled toward your spine, raise your head and shoulders off the floor. Pause for three seconds. Lower your head and shoulders. Do eight to 12 repetitions. Rest and repeat the set.

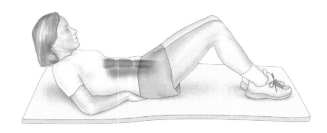

Power move: Lift your head and shoulders quickly off the floor. Hold briefly. Lower yourself at a normal pace. Do six to 10 repetitions.

If you have osteoporosis, talk to your doctor before trying this exercise. He or she may recommend that you avoid it.

9 Side bridge

Exercises the muscles of the shoulders, back, buttocks, and abdomen

Lie in a straight line on your left side on a mat. Bend both knees at a 90° angle so that your calves and feet point behind you. Raise your upper body, supporting it on the side of your left forearm. (Your left elbow should be bent at a 90° angle directly below your shoulder, and your forearm should point forward.) Now you are in the starting position. Slowly lift both hips a few inches upward to create a bridge until only your left forearm, knee, calf, and foot are touching the mat. Your spine should be in a neutral position (so it's in a straight line and isn't curved or arched). Pause. Lower yourself to the starting position. Do eight to 12 repetitions. Repeat on your right side. Rest and repeat the set.

Harder variation: Assume the starting position, but keep your legs straight. You can put your right leg behind your left leg to steady yourself, if you like. Once you are ready, slowly lift both hips a few inches upward to create a bridge until only your left forearm and foot are touching the mat. Pause. Lower yourself to the starting position. Do eight to 12 repetitions. Repeat on your right side. Rest and repeat the set.

Power move: Lift yourself quickly off the floor. Hold briefly. Lower yourself at a normal pace. Do six to 10 repetitions.

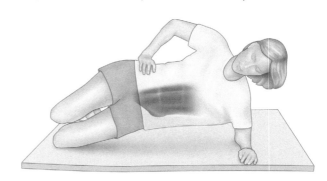

10 Back extension

Exercises the muscles of the back, hips, and buttocks

Find a sturdy counter that reaches about waist level. Face it, standing a couple of feet away. Distance yourself so that when you lean against the counter your body is at an angle of about 30° to 45°. Keeping your body straight and your arms across your chest (as if you are hugging yourself), lean forward so that you are resting your weight against the counter. Work up to holding for one minute. Rest and repeat for another set. (While most exercises in this workout are performed eight to 12 times in a set, this exercise is only done once per set.)

Harder variation: If you wish to push yourself further, you can work up to holding this position for two minutes, rather than one. Or instead of keeping your arms crossed during the move, reach your right arm up above your head so it is in a straight line with your torso and extend your left leg backward, raising it just an inch or two off the floor. Hold for 30 to 45 seconds. Then switch your arms and legs (lift your left arm and extend your right leg) and repeat. ◗

Harder variation

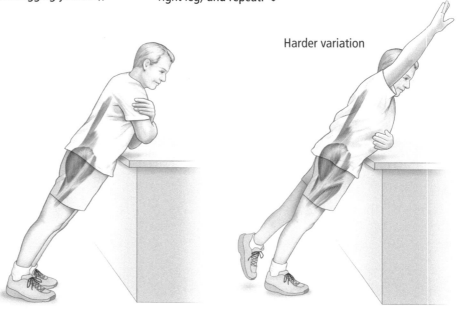

Balancing and stretching exercises

A complete exercise program should also include some balance and flexibility exercises. Adding these into your routine needn't be difficult or time-consuming. As you'll see, your current routine may already include some balance-improving exercises.

Stretching is also an important, if frequently over-looked, part of a routine. Note that the stretches shown in this chapter can also serve as your cool-down after strength training or aerobic activity.

Balancing

Several of the strength training exercises provided in Workout I and Workout II also help improve balance. So if you're regularly performing exercises such as the standing calf raise (page 32), chair stand (page 32), hip extension (page 33), and side leg raise (page 38), you may already be doing all you need to keep yourself steady on your feet. But if you aren't performing these exercises regularly or if you would like to further

Balancing and stretching exercises

1 Calf stretch

Stretches the Achilles tendon and calf

Stand in front of a wall with your palms flat against the wall and your elbows almost straight. Bend your right knee slightly, and step back a foot or two with your left leg, keeping the heel and foot flat on the floor and the feet pointing straight ahead. Hold for up to 30 seconds. You should feel this stretch in your calf and Achilles tendon; if you don't feel a stretch, move your foot back a bit farther. Switch legs and repeat.

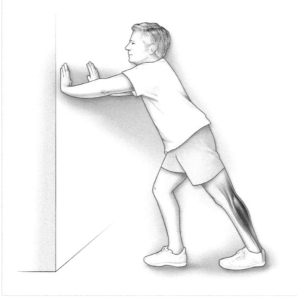

2 Quadriceps stretch

Stretches the front of the thigh

Steadying yourself with your left hand on a wall, stand with your feet together. Keeping the left leg straight, bend your right knee and grasp your ankle to pull your heel up toward your buttock. (You can wrap a belt or towel around your foot and pull on that if you are having trouble reaching your ankle.) Hold for up to 30 seconds. Switch legs and repeat.

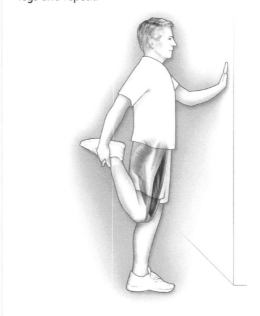

enhance your balance, you may want to try the following two exercises. These can be done anytime—every day of the week or just a few times a week.

Heel-to-toe walk

Position your heel just in front of the toes of the opposite foot each time you take a step. Heel and toes should actually touch as you walk forward for eight to 12 steps. If necessary, steady yourself by putting one hand on a counter as you walk at first, and then work toward doing this without support. Repeat two to four times.

Single-leg stance

Stand on one foot for up to 30 seconds. Put your foot down and rebalance yourself, then repeat on the opposite leg. Perform two to four times on each leg. If this is too difficult, you can steady yourself by holding on to the back of a chair or a counter at first. Then work toward doing this without support.

Stretching

Experts disagree about whether stretching prevents injury, mainly because there is a lack of hard evidence to this effect. We do know, however, that shorter, stiffer muscle fibers, which are an unfortunate result of getting older, may make you vulnerable to injuries. This can happen either because bones and joints are more easily pulled out of alignment, or simply because

3 Hamstring stretch

Stretches the back of the thigh

Stand behind a chair and hold the back of it with both hands. Walk your feet back and bend forward at your hips until your torso is parallel to the floor, feet under your hips. Lift your tailbone toward the ceiling to feel a deeper stretch down the back of your thighs. Try to keep your back and shoulders straight. Hold the position for up to 30 seconds.

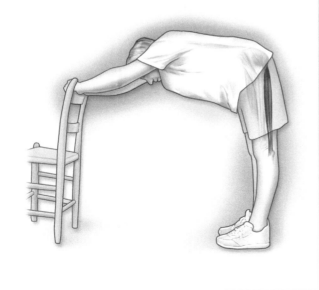

4 Double hip rotation*

Stretches the back and hips

Lie on your back with your knees bent and feet flat on the floor. Extend your arms out to the sides, palms up. Keep your shoulders on the floor throughout the exercise. Gently lower both legs to the left, keeping your knees together, and turn your head to the right. You should feel this stretch along the muscles of your hip, side, and, to a lesser extent, neck. Hold for up to 30 seconds. Bring your knees back to center and repeat on the other side.

*If you have osteoporosis or have had a hip replacement, talk to your doctor before trying this stretch. He or she may recommend that you avoid it.

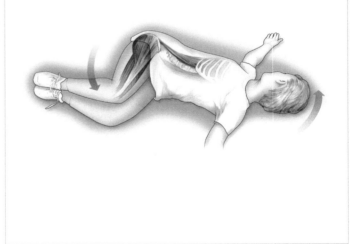

a tight muscle is more likely to tear under stress than one that is more flexible. We also know that when done correctly, stretching helps loosen tight muscles, keeping you more limber. It also gives you a greater, more comfortable range of motion and improves posture and balance.

So, regardless of whether there is proof that stretching actually prevents injury, it is an important part of overall musculoskeletal health. Experts used to recommend stretching before exercising, but newer research suggests that the best time to stretch is after exercising, as part of your cool-down session, because that is when muscles are most pliable. Stretching during your workout is fine, too, and may help boost flexibility.

Performing the stretches

Once your muscles are warmed up, you can do these 10 stretches anytime during the course of your workout. Some people like to do a stretch or two after each

5 Hip flexor stretch

Stretches the hip

Stand facing a chair, with the back of the chair against a wall for support. Raise your left foot up and rest it flat on the chair, with your knee bent. (Or you may prefer to place your foot on a stairstep, so that you can hold the railing for balance.) Keeping your spine as neutral as possible, press your pelvis forward gently until you feel a stretch at the top of the right thigh. Your pelvis will move forward only a little; the movement is subtle. Hold for up to 30 seconds. Repeat on the other side.

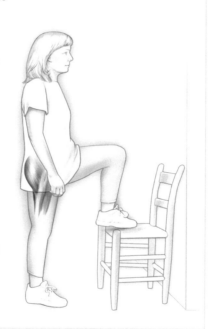

6 Side stretch

Stretches the side, shoulder, and arm

Stand or sit up in a chair. Reach upward with your left hand as far as you can while letting your right hand slide gently downward. You should feel this stretch along your rib cage, trunk, and waist. Hold for up to 30 seconds. Switch sides and repeat.

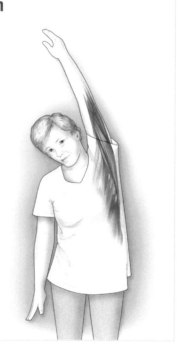

7 Shoulder rotation

Stretches the upper back, upper chest, and shoulders

Lie on your back on a mat with a pillow under your head. Stretch your legs out straight, or put a rolled towel beneath your knees if that's more comfortable. Extend your arms straight out to the sides, then bend your elbows 90° so your forearms are perpendicular to the floor and your hands are pointing toward the ceiling. Your shoulders and upper arms should remain flat on the mat. Now slowly lower your hands and forearms toward the floor by your head. Stop when you feel a stretch in your shoulders. Hold for up to 30 seconds. Raise your forearms slowly until your hands are pointing back at the ceiling. Now lower your bent arms in the opposite direction, forward toward the floor. Again stop when you feel a stretch in your shoulders. Hold for up to 30 seconds.

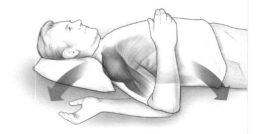

exercise; others prefer to stretch as part of their cool-down. Whichever you choose, be sure to hold each stretch for 10 to 30 seconds and repeat it for a total of one minute. If you hold the position for less time or do fewer repetitions, you won't lengthen the muscle fibers as effectively. On the other hand, holding a stretch for too long can increase your chances of injuring the muscle. When you are starting out, you may find that it's useful to time your stretches.

Here are some other safety tips:

- While stretching, remember to breathe normally.
- Don't bounce.
- Don't overextend your body. Stretch only to the point of mild tension, never pain. If a stretch hurts, stop immediately.
- If you have had a joint replaced or repaired, ask your surgeon whether you need to avoid certain stretches, such as the double hip rotation. If you have osteoporosis, consult your doctor before doing floor stretches or stretches that bend the spine.

Balancing and stretching exercises

8 Hip and lower back stretch*

Stretches the hips and lower back

Lie flat on your back with both legs extended. Keep your head on the floor, but look down toward your chest. Bend both knees and clasp them with your hands, pulling your knees toward your chest as far as is comfortable. Breathe in deeply and exhale, bringing the knees closer as you breathe out. You will feel compression in your hips and a stretch in your lower back. Hold for up to 30 seconds.

If you've had a hip replacement, check with your doctor before doing this stretch.

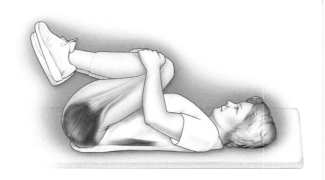

9 Inner leg stretch

Stretches the inner thigh

Sit on a mat with your knees bent and pointing outward, and your feet together. Draw your feet close to your body. Holding your shins or feet with your hands, bend your upper body forward and press your knees down with your elbows. Hold for up to 30 seconds.

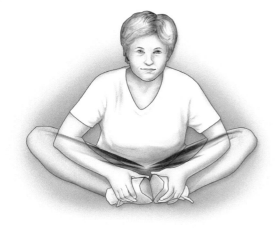

10 Triceps stretch

Stretches the triceps, rotator cuff, and upper back

Bend your right arm behind your neck, pointing your elbow toward the ceiling. Grasp your elbow with your left hand. Pull the raised right elbow gently toward the left until you feel a mild stretch at the back of your right upper arm. Hold for up to 30 seconds. Repeat with left arm.

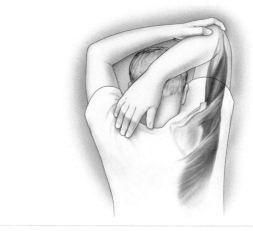

Strength training over a lifetime: Keys to staying motivated

Seeing results can be one of the biggest motivators for success with any behavior change, whether you are trying to lose weight, exercise more often, or quit smoking. The satisfaction you derive from seeing how your new behaviors have begun to affect your health—or your waist size—can entice you to keep going even if you are growing tired of the same old routine. However, in order to make strength and power training a lifelong endeavor, it's also a good idea to vary your routine and crank up the degree of challenge so you keep it fun and fresh.

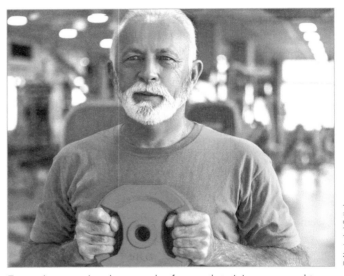

© Nastasic | Getty Images

To continue reaping the rewards of strength training, you need to keep doing it. Seeing results can help motivate you not to slack off.

Charting your progress

Probably the best way to keep track of your progress is to test yourself over time. Start by getting a baseline reading before you start the workouts in this report; then repeat the tests monthly, recording your results in the "Progress chart" on page 45. This written record can provide encouragement and help you stay motivated, because you'll see steady improvement if you stick to the program.

The National Institute on Aging recommends testing not only strength, but also endurance, lower-body power, and balance. Because strength and power training affect all of these—and a well-rounded exercise plan addresses the full quartet—the tests suggested in the chart should provide a good snapshot of your progress from one month to the next.

The chart has space for you to write down a few personal goals:

Why do you wish to do strength and power training? Are you hoping to tone your muscles? Boost energy? Or simply be able to heft your own groceries or walk easily up a flight or two of stairs? Reviewing your goals can help to keep you in the game when motivation starts to wane, providing additional reasons to keep going beyond simply charting improvements from month to month.

Continued on page 46

Progress chart

ACTIVITY	BASELINE	ONE MONTH	TWO MONTHS	THREE MONTHS	FOUR MONTHS
	Date: _____	Date: _____	Date: _____	Date: _____	Date: _____
Strength: Biceps curl (page 34) Write down the weight lifted and number of sets and reps of biceps curls you are able to do with each arm.	Weight: _____ Sets: _____ Reps: (R) _____ Reps: (L) _____	Weight: _____ Sets: _____ Reps: (R) _____ Reps: (L) _____	Weight: _____ Sets: _____ Reps: (R) _____ Reps: (L) _____	Weight: _____ Sets: _____ Reps: (R) _____ Reps: (L) _____	Weight: _____ Sets: _____ Reps: (R) _____ Reps: (L) _____
Strength: Chair stand (page 32) Time how long it takes to do 10 chair stands. Aim to do the exercise without using your arms to help. If you need to use your arms, check "arms"; otherwise, check "no arms." Be sure to exercise at a safe pace and use good form.	Time: _____ ☐ Arms ☐ No arms	Time: _____ ☐ Arms ☐ No arms	Time: _____ ☐ Arms ☐ No arms	Time: _____ ☐ Arms ☐ No arms	Time: _____ ☐ Arms ☐ No arms
Lower-body power Time yourself as you go up a flight of at least 10 stairs, then walk down it at your usual pace. If that seems way too easy from the start, try going up and down the stairs two or three times or doing more than one flight. Just be sure to use the same number of flights or stairs each month. Number of flights or stairs: _____	Time: _____	Time: _____	Time: _____	Time: _____	Time: _____
Balance Time how long you can stand unsupported on one foot. Do this for each foot.	Left: _____ Right: _____	Left: _____ Right: _____	Left: _____ Right: _____	Left: _____ Right: _____	Left: _____ Right: _____
Endurance Time how long it takes you to walk four blocks or another specific distance. Use the same course each time.	Time: _____	Time: _____	Time: _____	Time: _____	Time: _____
Personal goals	Changes	Changes	Changes	Changes	Changes
1.					
2.					
3.					
4.					

Continued from page 44

How soon can you expect to see gains? Research suggests the biggest gains occur within the first four to eight weeks of strength and power training. After that, you should still progress, but most likely at a slower pace.

This chart covers five months. If you copy the blank chart, you can continue testing yourself after that, too. Write in the month and day of each set of tests, the results of the tests, and changes you've observed in your abilities. Try to check your progress on the same day of each month and at the same time of day, if possible, for the most comparable results.

Stepping up the pace

Because your body adapts to whatever demands you regularly place upon it, you must gradually make your workout more difficult in order to continue improving your fitness. This can also keep you challenged and interested in your fitness routine. You are ready to increase the challenge whenever your current regimen becomes too easy to accomplish. There are several ways to do this:

Add repetitions. Aim for the maximum of 12 repetitions; after that, increase weight.

Add a set. Perform three or four sets of each exercise instead of two. After that, increase the weight or change another parameter, such as repetitions or exercises.

Add weight. This is an easy change to make—up to a point. If you're using ankle weights for lower-body work, you may need to do additional exercises to make further gains, or you might need to switch to machines, which will allow you to use heavier leg weights (more than 20 pounds). When you add weight, drop back to two sets if you have been doing three or four, until that seems too easy. For power training, you can also try a weighted vest (see "How to use a weighted vest," at left).

Add exercises. If you are performing Workout I, you may want to add a few exercises from Workout II to make your routine longer. If you are already doing Workout II, you can add some exercises from "Moving onward: Switching up your routine" on page 49.

How to use a weighted vest

If you want to wear a weighted vest when doing some of the power moves described in this report—notably, the standing calf raise (page 32), chair stand (page 32), stair climbing (page 33), triceps dip (page 34), bridge (page 38), and side bridge (page 39)—choose one that can hold a total of 7 to 25 pounds in half-pound to 1-pound bars. The maximum amount of weight you use in your vest depends on your body weight. The chart here can help you determine the upper limit that's right for you.

Begin by wearing the vest without any weights. After two to three workouts with just the vest, add weight in the amount described in the chart. Increase the weights every week or two, in the same increments. Once the total reaches the upper limit set for your body weight, stop adding weights.

For example, a 120-pound woman would add 2 pounds to her vest every week or two. Over the course of about six to 12 weeks, the weight would increase as follows: the vest alone, 2 pounds, 4 pounds, 6 pounds, 8 pounds, 10 pounds, and finally 12 pounds. She should not put more than 12 pounds into her vest.

If your workout feels too vigorous at any time or if you can't complete the recommended two to three sets of an exercise with the vest on, reduce the amount of weight in your vest to a more comfortable level.

Guidelines for adding weight to your vest

IF YOU WEIGH:	INCREASE THE WEIGHT AT REGULAR INTERVALS BY THIS AMOUNT	MAXIMUM AMOUNT TO USE IN YOUR VEST
75–99 pounds	1 pound	7 pounds
100–149 pounds	2 pounds	12 pounds
150–199 pounds	3 pounds	18 pounds
200–239 pounds	4 pounds	20 pounds
240–280 pounds	5 pounds	25 pounds

Keeping it interesting

If you feel yourself balking at the thought of one more day of the same old routine or find you've reached a plateau, consider making some changes. The following suggestions can help you add variety to your workout.

Mix it up. Vary your program by switching the order in which you do the exercises. Although committed bodybuilders deliberately move in sequence from larger muscles to smaller muscles, the rest of us needn't follow such an absolute order.

Make substitutions. You can swap exercises that focus on strengthening the same basic muscle groups. That is, choose a different exercise that works leg muscles or upper arm muscles. You can use the examples found in "Moving onward: Switching up your routine" (page 49) or get ideas from other publications on strength training, as well as exercise videos and classes.

Change your pace. Vary the intensity of your workouts. For example, do one hard, one medium, and one lighter workout in cycles of seven to 10 days. This is a form of periodization—an exercise strategy that can enhance strength gains, help sidestep boredom and plateaus, and prevent overtraining while allowing more time for the body to heal after being thoroughly taxed. Reps, sets, and resistance for different exercises are varied to achieve these

Vary your equipment

Variety adds spice to all parts of life, and working out is no different. These strengthening tools can help you avoid becoming complacent or bored. Talk with a personal trainer about whether they're right for you.

Medicine balls are used for core, strength, and power exercises. They are about the size of a soccer ball and come in a variety of weights. You can lift or toss them to work your muscles in new ways.

Resistance bands look like big, wide rubber bands and come in several levels of resistance, designated by color. You can use bands in place of dumbbells for some exercises, such as biceps curls or overhead presses, or do other exercises specifically designed for resistance bands. Bands provide more resistance on the eccentric contraction than dumbbells.

Resistance tubing comes in several levels of resistance, also coded by color. Look for tubing with padded handles on each end. Some brands come with a doorknob attachment helpful for anchoring the tubing in place when doing certain exercises. Resistance tubing works like a resistance band, but it is more durable. The handles can make it easier to use, especially if you have arthritis in your hands.

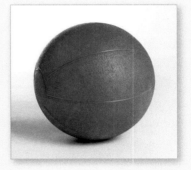

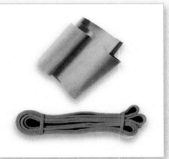

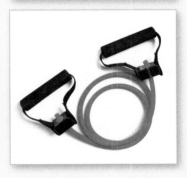

goals. Because it can be difficult to put together a good periodization strategy, it's essential to work with an exercise professional to come up with a plan that's right for you.

Work out with a friend when you can. If your friend is careful about good form, too, this can be a way to help reinforce good habits. Some gyms have a buddy board to help members find workout partners.

Join a class. The camaraderie and supervision can be helpful. Plus, you'll probably learn something new.

Work with a trainer. Pay for a session or two with a certified personal trainer who can help you develop a well-rounded new routine.

Put on music that raises your spirits. Music has been shown to inspire exercisers to work out

© claudiahung | Getty Images

© Sovos | Getty Images

© herreid | Getty Images

harder, which helps explain why gyms always play music for exercise classes. If you need more of a distraction, you could watch a favorite TV show while you exercise once you've mastered the moves.

Try new equipment. Substitute one type of equipment for another if you belong to a gym that offers a good range. For example, try working out with machines instead of free weights one day a week or switching from one brand of machine to another. Or you might try new exercises using a medicine ball, resistance bands, or resistance tubing. (See "Vary your equipment" on page 47 for more detailed descriptions.) A good trainer can help.

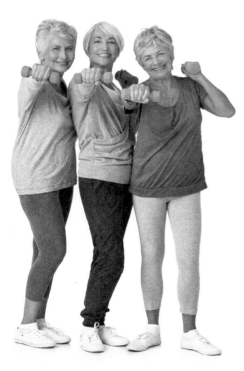

Working out with friends can help keep you motivated. It's more fun that way—and you're less likely to cancel out.

Shoring up motivation

Usually, we do our best work when motivated. That extends to exercise, too. It's not uncommon to launch a new exercise program raring to go, only to wind up back on the couch with your feet propped up just a few weeks later. If your will wavers in spite of the gains in your monthly progress chart, try these tips.

Refresh your memory. Remind yourself how the exercises will help you by reading your goals again. Emphasize the positive aspects of your new routine. Rather than sternly saying, "I should do my workout," say "I feel so much better when I do strength and power exercises" or "I can accomplish my daily tasks more easily when I do my workout."

Find the time. All too often, the reason we don't exercise is that we "don't have time." If that's true for you, try grabbing pockets of down time throughout the day and using those for some strength and power moves. While you're on the phone, for example, do 10 chair stands. Keep some light hand weights in your living room, and do some biceps curls while you watch TV, or some triceps dips during commercial breaks. You may be able to squeeze an entire workout into your day by breaking it up.

Find a workout buddy. Workouts with a friend or family member are more fun, plus you're less likely to cancel on the spur of the moment if someone else is holding you accountable. If finding a workout partner isn't possible, ask a friend or relative to check in with you on a regular basis—on workout days or maybe just once a week—to give you a pat on the back or a pep talk.

Plan simple rewards. Give yourself a small reward for every success, big or small. Treat yourself to something you would like—a cup of coffee with a friend, a small square of your favorite chocolate, a movie. Be creative.

Maintaining gains

Muscles stay strong with regular workouts, but the gains slip away quickly if those workouts stop. To keep building strength and power and to achieve the fullest gains possible, continue training for two or three days a week.

At some point, though, that may not be possible. You may get busy and be able to fit in only one session a week. You may need to cut back during a vacation or for a longer period of time—for example, if you're sick. Remember that doing something is better than nothing. You could break up your workout and do one or two exercises a day instead of trying to do them all on the same day. You can also try to fit in some other activities, depending upon your situation. This can help you stay in good shape and lead a healthy, active, and independent life. And as soon as possible, get back to your regular routine.

© Cecilie_Arcurs | Getty Images

Moving onward: Switching up your routine

You can freshen up a stale routine by substituting exercises that target the same basic muscles. Here are just a few options to get you started.

Thigh raise

Exercises the muscles of the hips and front thighs

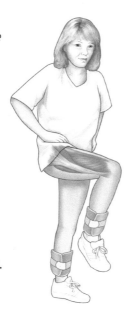

Wearing ankle weights, stand with your hands on your hips. Keeping your back straight, raise your knee up until your thigh is parallel to the floor (your foot will be lifted off the floor). Pause. Lower the leg to the starting position. Do eight to 12 repetitions. Repeat with the opposite leg. This is one complete set. Rest and repeat the set.

Easier variation: Stand next to a chair and hold on to the back of it for balance, if necessary. Raise the knee that's farthest away from the chair up to hip height. Pause. Lower the leg. Do eight to 12 repetitions. Rest and repeat the set. Then turn your other side to the chair and repeat with your other leg.

Power move: Lift your leg quickly. Hold briefly. Lower your leg at a normal pace. Do six to 10 repetitions.

Knee flexor

Exercises the back thigh muscles

Wearing ankle weights, stand behind a chair with your hands on the back of it. Bend one knee to bring your foot close to the back of your thigh, keeping your back straight and your upper leg as still as possible. Pause. Lower the leg to the starting position and repeat with the opposite leg. Do eight to 12 repetitions. Rest and repeat the set.

Power move: Lift your lower leg quickly. Hold briefly. Lower your leg at a normal pace. Do six to 10 repetitions.

Knee squeeze

Exercises the inner thigh muscles

On a mat, lie on your back with your knees bent and your feet flat on the floor. Place a ball about the size of a soccer ball between your knees. Squeeze your thighs together as hard as you can for a count of three. Release and repeat. Do eight to 12 repetitions. Rest and repeat the set.

Harder variation: Do this exercise standing. Simply place the ball between your knees and squeeze hard for three seconds.

Power move: Squeeze and release as quickly as possible. Do six to 10 repetitions.

Push-up

Exercises the muscles of the chest and back upper arms

On a mat, balance on your hands and the balls of your feet and toes, holding your body straight with your palms flat on the mat, hands directly under your shoulders, and elbows slightly bent. Your feet may be together or a bit apart. Keeping your body in line from head to heels, bend your elbows out to the sides and lower your body toward the floor without touching the mat. Then push yourself back upward until your arms are extended, without locking your elbows. Do eight to 12 repetitions. Rest and repeat the set.

Easier variations: If a full push-up is too challenging, try knee push-ups, balancing your weight on your knees instead of your toes. Or do wall push-ups: Stand up straight in front of a wall with your arms extended at shoulder height, palms against the wall, and your fingers pointing upward. Bend your elbows to bring your upper body as close to the wall as possible. Pause. Push away from the wall to return to the starting position, keeping your body in line from head to heels throughout the movement. Do eight to 12 repetitions. Rest and repeat the set.

Power move: Lower at a normal pace, hold briefly, and then press up quickly. Do six to 10 repetitions.

Moving onward: Switching up your routine *continued*

Opposite arm and leg raise

Exercises the muscles of the buttocks, spine, and shoulders

On a mat, get down on your hands and knees. Look down at the floor, keeping your neck straight. Exhale as you slowly extend your right leg and left arm. Keep your back flat while doing this. Pause. Inhale as you return to the starting position. Do eight to 12 repetitions. Repeat with your left leg and right arm. Rest and repeat the set.

Power move: Lift your arm and leg quickly. Hold briefly. Lower at a normal pace. Do six to 10 repetitions.

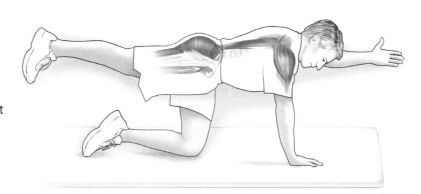

Upright row

Exercises the muscles of the shoulders, upper back, and front upper arms

Stand with your feet shoulder-width apart. With your arms at your sides, hold a dumbbell in each hand. Your palms should be facing your thighs. Bend your elbows out to the sides and slowly lift both dumbbells straight up to chest or shoulder height, whichever is more comfortable. As you lift, keep the weights close to your body. Pause. Slowly lower the dumbbells back down to your thighs. Do eight to 12 repetitions. Rest and repeat the set.

Power move: Lift your arms quickly. Hold briefly. Lower at a normal pace. Do six to 10 repetitions. ◥

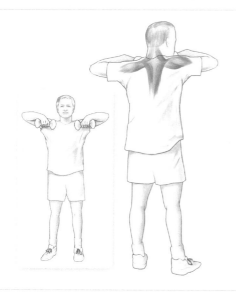

Resources

Organizations

American Academy of Physical Medicine and Rehabilitation
9700 W. Bryn Mawr Ave., Suite 200
Rosemont, IL 60018
847-737-6000
www.aapmr.org

This national organization is for doctors who specialize in physical medicine and rehabilitation for musculoskeletal and neurological problems. A referral service on the website can help you locate physiatrists in your area.

American College of Sports Medicine
401 W. Michigan St.
Indianapolis, IN 46206
317-637-9200
www.acsm.org

ACSM is a nonprofit that educates and certifies fitness professionals, such as personal trainers, and offers information to the public on strength and power training and other types of exercise. A referral service on the website (www.acsm.org/get-stay-certified/find-a-pro) lists ACSM-certified personal trainers.

American Council on Exercise
4851 Paramount Drive
San Diego, CA 92123
888-825-3636 (toll-free)
www.acefitness.org

ACE is a nonprofit organization that promotes fitness and offers a wide array of educational materials for consumers and professionals. The website includes a library of free exercise videos and a referral service to locate ACE-certified personal trainers and health coaches.

American Physical Therapy Association
1111 N. Fairfax St.
Alexandria, VA 22314
800-999-2782 (toll-free)
www.apta.org

This national professional organization fosters advances in education, research, and the practice of physical therapy. Its consumer website (www.moveforwardPT.com) provides information on how physical therapy can help a variety of conditions, gives patient stories, and includes a search engine to locate board-certified physical therapists in your area.

Arthritis Foundation
1355 Peachtree St. NE, Suite 600
Atlanta, GA 30309
800-283-7800 (toll-free)
www.arthritis.org

This nonprofit organization offers free publications on many arthritic conditions as well as information on exercise, research, and current treatments.

National Institute on Aging
Building 31, Room 5C27
31 Center Drive, MSC 2292
Bethesda, MD 20892

800-222-2225 (toll-free)
www.go4life.nia.nih.gov

Part of the National Institutes of Health, the National Institute on Aging has a physical activity campaign, called Go4Life. Its website offers exercises, motivational tips, and free resources to help older adults get ready, start exercising, and keep going.

Special Health Reports

The following Special Health Reports from Harvard Medical School will give you more exercises to expand your program in different ways. Order online at www.health.harvard.edu or call 877-649-9457 (toll-free).

Better Balance: Simple exercises to improve stability and prevent falls
Suzanne Salamon, M.D., and Brad Manor, Ph.D., Medical Editors
(Harvard Medical School, 2017)

Gradual changes linked to growing older—such as weak or inflexible muscles, slower reflexes, and worsening eyesight—can erode your sense of balance. This report provides six complete workouts, starting with a beginner balance workout and progressing through more advanced exercises to help prevent falls, build better awareness of your body, boost your confidence, and keep you healthy and independent.

Gentle Core Exercises: Start toning your abs, building your back muscles, and reclaiming core fitness today
Lauren E. Elson, M.D., Medical Editor, with Michele Stanten, Fitness Consultant
(Harvard Medical School, 2017)

Want to bring more power to pursuits like swimming, golf, and tennis? Ward off or ease lower back pain? Build up your balance and stability so that you're less likely to fall? A strong, flexible core underpins all these goals. If you need to approach core work gently—perhaps because you've been ill or you're afraid of aggravating an injury—this report can provide solutions. Includes exercises that can be done at the office.

Starting to Exercise
Lauren E. Elson, M.D., Medical Editor, with Michele Stanten, Fitness Consultant
(Harvard Medical School, 2018)

This report takes you through a complete program of exercise, including aerobic training, walking workouts, strength training, and more. If you've never had a formal exercise program—or you've allowed your exercise routine to lapse over the years—this report will show you how to start rebuilding your fitness.

Stretching: 35 stretches to improve flexibility and reduce pain
Lauren E. Elson, Medical Editor, with Michele Stanten, Fitness Consultant
(Harvard Medical School, 2017)

Stretching can help prevent or relieve stiffness, improve sports performance, and, in older adults, make daily activities easier. This report includes stretches you can do while lying on the floor, seated in a chair, or standing.

Glossary

aerobic activity: An activity or exercise that increases heart rate and breathing through repetitive use of large muscles, such as walking, running, or biking. Also known as endurance or cardio exercise, aerobic activity conditions the heart, lungs, circulatory system, and muscles.

concentric contraction: When muscles exert force and move joints by shortening.

eccentric contraction: When muscles exert force and move joints by lengthening.

fast-twitch fiber: One of two main types of skeletal muscle fibers. Fast-twitch fibers are recruited most heavily when bursts of power are needed, as in sprinting.

isometric (static) contraction: When muscles generate force, but neither contract nor extend enough to move a joint (such as when someone pushes against an immovable object).

motor unit: The pairing of a nerve cell and the group of muscle fibers it commands.

muscle fibers: Cells bundled together to make up muscle tissue.

myofibrils: Long interlocking strands that make up muscle fibers.

myofilaments: The fundamental muscle proteins that form myofibrils. Myofilaments slide over one another, bunching up and generating force, when a muscle contracts.

periodization: An exercise strategy that varies reps, sets, and resistance to alternate heavier and lighter workouts over a period of time.

power: Force times speed of movement. It reflects how quickly a force is exerted.

power training: An emerging field of physical medicine aimed at boosting the ability to exert strength quickly, especially in relation to practical, day-to-day tasks.

repetitions ("reps"): The number of times an exercise calls for a muscle to be worked and released (usually eight to 12).

set: A given number of repetitions of an exercise.

skeletal muscles: Muscles attached to bones throughout the body that allow voluntary movement to occur.

slow-twitch fiber: One of two main types of skeletal muscle fibers. Slow-twitch fibers are recruited most heavily for endurance (aerobic) exercises.

specificity: Activities that target the specific muscles and moves needed for the tasks of daily life or a sport rather than for the sake of building muscles.

strength: The ability to exert force.

strength training: Popular term for exercises that harness resistance supplied by body weight, free weights such as dumbbells or weighted cuffs, or specialized machines. Also known as resistance training, progressive resistance training, or weight training.

tendon: A cord of connective tissue tethered at one end to muscle and at the other end to bone.